DRESS
FOR
EXCELLENCE

DRESS

FOR

EXCELLENCE

———

Lois Fenton

with Edward Olcott

RAWSON ASSOCIATES · New York

Rawson Associates
Macmillan Publishing Comapny
866 Third Avenue, New York, NY 1022
Collier Macmillan Canada, Inc.

Library of Congress Cataloging-in-Publication Data
Fenton, Lois.
   Dress for excellence.

   Includes index.
   1. Men's clothing.   2. Grooming for men.   I. Olcott,
Edward.   II. Title.
TT617.F46 1986   646'.32   85-43086
ISBN 0-89256-304-4

Macmillan books are available at special discounts for bulk purchases for sales promotions, premiums, fund-raising, or educational use. For details, contact:

Special Sales Director
Macmillan Publishing Company
866 Third Avenue
New York, NY 10022

10 9 8 7 6 5 4 3 2
Designed by Jacques Chazaud
Illustrations by Al Hughes
Printed in the United States of America

Photographs by Amy Meadow, with the exception of the photograph of Don Johnson and Philip Michael Thomas, which is by Douglas Keeve/Gamma Liaison; the photograph of Ron Darling, which is copyright © by George Kalinsky; and the photographs of George L. Ball, Paul H. Pearson (copyright © 1985 by Burlingame), and Kenneth C. Nichols.

To my mother,
who taught me to love wonderful clothes,
and my father,
who was obsessed with excellence.
And to my four sons,
Kirk, Gregg, Scott, and Matt,
who made it clear to me that
each man is an individual,
different from his brothers.

Contents

Acknowledgements

I want to thank the many people who helped me turn a series of lectures and an idea into the book *Dress for Excellence*. My grateful appreciation to:

Toni Sciarra for her intelligent and insightful editing;

My literary agents, Connie Clausen and Guy Kettelhack;

Amy Meadow for her impeccable judgment and her distinctive photographs;

Al Hughes, for his artistic—and accurate—drawings;

My friends, the listeners, Marlene Schechtman and Phyllis Adler;

Brian Stewart, for his unerring eye and his knowledgeable advice;

My brother Howard, sister Nancy, and their spouses and my friends, Elaine and Bob, for continuing to be there for me;

A dear old friend, Libby R. K. Isaac, whose suggestion years ago piqued me into my lecturing career;

Two old friends, Lester and Bob, for cheering me on;

Seymour Levine, for his adult approach and his uncommon way with words;

The people who contributed their invaluable time, help, and counsel: Sidney Albert, G. Chris Andersen, William P. Archer, Arthur Ashe, Jr., George L. Ball, Roger Baugh, Dan Berg, Michael D. Brown, John Carter, Eugene Cernan, Sherry Suib Cohen, Richard Cyert, Ron Darling, William Dill, Marvin Feldman, Andrew Fezza, Donald M. Fordyce, Bernie Goldsmith, Eugene Grant, Robert Green, Arthur Grodd, Joseph Guiffre, Clara Hancox, Kevin Harrington, Elliot M. Hershberg, Arthur Hettich, Jay Horwitz, Jack Hyde, Carol Jenkins, Frederick H. Joseph, John H. Kissick, Smitty Kogan, Matthew Kornreich, Morton Kornreich, Richard Kove, Paul Kovi, Wilbert J. LeMelle, James Mainwood, Stanley Marcus, Tom Margittai, Hans Mark, Thomas McAboy, Robert A. Meister, Ken Nichols, Lilian Owen, Paul H. Pearson, Bert Pulitzer, Corrine Pulitzer, James D. Robinson, III, Chuck Scarborough, Bud Schiff, John Schornack, John Silton, Allan Tessler, Frank Walton;

Matt Fenton, my personal organizer and ongoing editor, for all of his tremendous help and specifically for his major contribution to Chapter 17;

Especially Sidney Gerhardt, who taught me to have faith in myself;

And, of course, the thousands of men who have attended my Executive Wardrobe Engineering seminars, who have responded so openly and enthusiastically, and prompted me to write *Dress for Excellence*.

1

What This Book Will Tell You

There Is No Erase Button

At an initial meeting, you form your first impression of someone largely on appearance—usually in the first forty seconds! You don't yet know his IQ or his theories about reducing the deficit. What you do know is how he looks—how he *dresses* and how much authority he seems to possess.

In a group of a dozen executives, there is always one whom you will immediately recognize as the person in charge. He has the look, the feel, the assertion of power.

And in the same way that you form a judgment, the world judges you. First impressions are lasting ones. *There is no erase button.*

We would like to think that we have open minds—that we revise our first opinions after we get to know someone. If he is brighter than he seemed, or indispensable to the

corporate welfare, he'll move up in our rating file. But it happens rarely—
and slowly.

It Could Happen . . .

You have an appointment with a key vice-president of one of the
largest companies in the city. You're part of a four-member committee concerned with a public service matter, an important community
issue. The other three men are in your salary range: high. They are
about your age.

You feel uncomfortable, slightly at a disadvantage. You feel that
you're an outsider. This is the third meeting, and it has been this way
every time.

At the first meeting you were wearing your dark brown suit. It's
a perfectly respectable suit, or was when you bought it two years
ago. It cost $225 then and prices have gone up since.

George and Peter were wearing dark blue suits, fine ones.
Bob's dark gray pinstripe was remarkable. Every thread, every
crease, was just right. His shirt was crisp—obviously ironed by a
professional. In fact, all three of them looked perfect. All you could
think was that brown was the wrong color. And probably that olive-
toned tie was a mistake, as well.

You suspect that all three formed an unspoken opinion of you
that afternoon and never changed it. You're probably right. After all,
they are no different about changing their minds than you are. When
was the last time you revised your opinion of someone you didn't
feel was first-rate?

My Promise to You

I am not going to tell you—and you've come too far to believe in rainbows
and pots of gold—that all you've got to do is get a $600 pinstriped navy
blue suit, a $50 shirt, and a $40 tie and you'll be Mr. Wonderful.

What I do promise you is a feeling of confidence, of belonging, that translates into *authority*. I see it wherever I go, and my background includes a lifetime of interest and involvement in clothes: six years in the Men's Division of Neiman-Marcus and more than ten years in professional teaching, consulting, and lecturing about executive wardrobe engineering. The men at the very top of my client firms—among whom are Arthur Young & Company, Drexel Burnham Lambert Incorporated, Metropolitan Life, J I Case, United States Steel, Carnegie-Mellon University, American Bankers Association, Coopers & Lybrand, and dozens of others—know that clothes are not indirect helpers; appearance translates *directly* into power.

When I speak at conferences, my seminar is usually the one program *not* based on the general subject of the meeting. Yet over the past few years my share of the audience has grown—from the early times when I hoped I would have a decent turnout to more recent times when mine is an embarrassment of riches—many more men attend my session than any of the technical topics. The other speakers are in small conference rooms, while I am speaking in the ballroom.

I do not claim the credit for this. The men who come to hear me do not know ahead of time how effective or interesting a speaker I will be. But men today are more openly interested in dress, and they are ready to come, listen, and learn. They, like you, understand how vital it is to look their best.

You have an untapped capacity to *extend your sphere of influence* over colleagues and customers, and once you begin to dress for excellence, that capacity will emerge.

Like John F. Akers, president and CEO of IBM, you will realize that *real* power gives you flexibility; you need not exercise it in expected ways. The story is told of his appearing for the first time at the offices of a large corporation IBM had just acquired. He wore a tan suit to demonstrate that IBM officers do not always wear blue "IBM uniform" suits, and to silently assure executives of the new company that they would not be molded into any pattern.

George Gobel, for my money one of the most perceptive humorists we've ever known, knows what it is to strive toward membership in the select, inside group. One evening George was a guest on the "Tonight Show" with Johnny Carson. He looked around at the other guests, all of whom were well dressed, and asked, "Have you ever felt that the whole world was a tuxedo and you were a pair of brown shoes?" The truth of the matter is this: The world is made of little cliques. Wearing the right clothes gets you into the top ones.

During the question periods after my talks, I've heard managers reveal their frustrations at not quite making the grade; at being treated cordially, but not truly accepted at the top levels and not given a high profile in the company.

When you have read this book, I know that you will be ready to *Dress for Excellence*. It happens because your perception of yourself catches up to reality. It is an aspect of what I call mirroring. Let me explain how it works.

Everyone has someone who represents the right way to look, the right way to walk. If you could do it all over, that's who you'd like to be. For John F. Kennedy, it was his brother Joe. For you, it might be Lee Iacocca or Senator Bill Bradley, or perhaps one of the top officers of your firm. Whoever it is, you inwardly compare yourself with that image. And since you've picked a high achiever, one who has risen over many others, you have set a lofty goal for yourself.

The first thing you've got to do is separate the fantasy from the reality. Of course, keep your goals high. But do it with the realization that you are distinctly, individually *you*. Perhaps your choice of clothes will reflect that of a role model or mentor, but you will want to add the individual touches that make you look not like someone else, but like *yourself* at *your* best.

Your appearance is truly the one factor you can control. If you package yourself to manage the impression you make on others, then their positive reinforcement will, in time, make you the person you want to be. You decide! It's up to you. If you want to be successful—look successful.

—WILLIAM THOURLBY,
You Are What You Wear

You're going to extract the very best from your present self. You're going to improve the hand that was dealt you, and play it to win.

In my talks with managers from almost every kind of background—those who have fought up the hard way or inherited their luck; those in smokestack industries, the professions, or the financial world—I have learned that there are two common obstacles to dressing for excellence, to living up to your full potential.

Obstacle 1—Guilt About Spending. A part of our American work ethic, probably an inheritance from those Puritans who were the first "no frills" consumers, is a deep-seated guilt about spending money on ourselves. It is vanity, we believe, or self-indulgence, or something equally loathsome. Nonsense. There's not a thing wrong with spending *more* than you ever thought decent to pay for suits, coats, shirts, and ties. The guilt comes about through uncertainty. "Is this really a good buy? Am I throwing away money?"

These doubts create anxiety, nervousness about the whole shopping experience; and in creeps the guilt. But once you *know* that you're getting more for your money, that your expensive new clothes are an investment that any informed, prudent executive would make, the guilt can subside. This book gives you the knowledge you need in order to make clothing purchases without a single twinge of doubt or guilt.

"What's your idea of looking good?" a writer for *The New York Times* asked several fashion authorities. Their answers:

Looking good is one of the finer pleasures in life. People have come around to openly believing that looking good is okay.
—BILL BLASS, designer

For most people, it really means looking like someone else, a perception created by an abstract other. . . . It's a metaphor for our inner being. . . . Society doesn't applaud people's looking bad. Looking bad means we feel bad about ourselves.
—CHARLES HIX, author

If you look good, my clothes support that in you. But looking good is feeling good, and feeling good is being at peace with yourself.
—PERRY ELLIS, designer

Obstacle 2—Fear of Style. It might take some self-probing to recognize it, but could there be a strain of *fear of style* in your personality? A reluctance to try a more elegant suit or one of the new fabrics, like pinpoint oxford cloth? Does the idea of wearing a splendid $70 Ralph Lauren shirt, updating your hairstyle, or tucking a silk foulard square in your breast pocket make you think, "Sounds great, but I don't think I could carry it off"?

Michael Korda, senior vice-president and editor in chief of Simon & Schuster and author of *Success!*, says that fear of fashion is far from rare, but that conquering it is far from difficult. "Dressing badly," he wrote in a *Playboy* article, "indicates a certain contempt for other people, which will be forgiven only if you are very rich or very talented or simply have no social, financial, or business ambitions." The essentials, he says, are simplicity and the courage to indulge your whims. Above all, know that class shows, class counts, and *class can be learned*.

How to Make Important People
Accept Your Importance

Successful people dress in a certain way. They respect others who do the same. Top men in industry seek out others who reflect themselves. The thinking is, "I'm an important person. I dress this way. If you dress this way, too, you're also important."

These men don't set down rules on how their people should dress. But it's human nature that they seek out those who reflect their image.

You might think that bucking the traditions asserts your independence and individuality. But in reality you are placing at risk your chances of top-level success in the business and business/social worlds as they exist today.

If you are motivated to dress for excellence, *this is the book for you*. On the pages that follow you will see living examples of many of our country's top executives who do just that. Their apparel—and their comments—are fascinating insights into attitudes at the top about personal style and appearance.

2

Leadership Looks – Advice from Executives Who Have Learned the Look of Command

Ihave mentioned my conviction that an *image* of confidence and authority begets *actual* authority and power. I learned it from observing and talking with scores of leaders in American life—business, government, the professions, sports, the academic world—men whose ability and drive to succeed carried them to the top.

I would like to share some of their thoughts on what it takes to get to the very top . . . and the part clothes play in that climb.

These extraordinary achievers have definite ideas about personal style and its impact on success. They should know. They are proof that it works. Insights into their attitudes about dress and image, combined with the rules and observations you will find in this book, give you a can't-miss formula for capitalizing on those attitudes.

Although some of these men have been clients of mine and others manage organizations where I have given my seminars, by no means is this the case with all those who generously gave their time to be photographed and interviewed for this book. I asked these men to agree to be in the book because each and every one possesses the unmistakable look of excellence that, combined with his prodigious accomplishments, stamps him as a leader in his field.

Some of the most revealing insights about what distinguishes certain men from all others came from my interview with George L. Ball, chairman and CEO of Prudential-Bache Securities, Inc.:

"Clothes do not make the man, but they are a way of stating his value codes. If you are dealing in a scarce commodity like money, appearances are a guide to the mind-set—the values—of the person you are conversing with.

"Early in my days on Wall Street, we were contemplating doing business with a certain company. When we met with them, two or three of their senior executives were dressed in suits with large patterns; they had almost a garish appearance. The decision was made not to finance that company. It was in part their general image that resulted in the 'no-go' decision."

Mr. Ball went on to define his own firm's corporate position on these matters. "Here at Prudential-Bache, we have a course in how to dress, and a tailor on the premises. We don't do this to dictate how people should dress, but we want them to feel at their best—and we know their time is limited. No matter what kind of suit a man wears, we want to be sure it is cut right and fits well."

Asked how men dress in the nation's capital, he answered: "You can tell a Senate staffer or a Ways and Means Committee aide-de-camp by the clothes he wears. Clothing becomes a surrogate for a label on the outside telling people who you are. As you move up the ranks to elected officialdom, you start to see variations: purposely countrified or studiously dandified. The young politicians with legal or business backgrounds are Paul Stuarted to the nines."

His reply when I asked him to comment on the relationship between dress and success was: "Generalizations in business are risky, but . . . people who present themselves extremely well are usually the ones who have the persistence, the drive, the ability, and the character to achieve success over a protracted period of time."

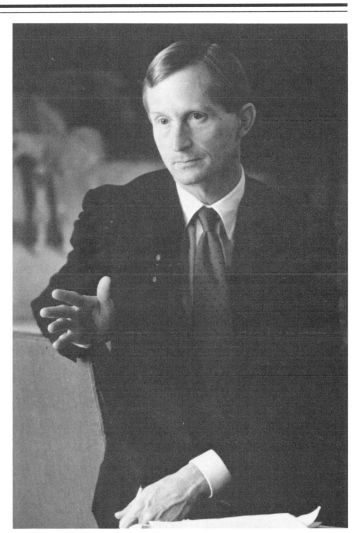

George L. Ball
executive

As chairman and CEO of Prudential-Bache Securities, George Ball exemplifies American leadership. The traditional elements—a fine dark blue pinstriped suit, white point-collar shirt, and bright red and navy polka-dot silk tie in a perfect four-in-hand knot—provide an effective contrast to his light hair and fair coloring.

A client firm I especially enjoy working with is Drexel Burnham Lambert Incorporated, one of the nation's outstanding financial organizations. It is an ongoing pleasure to advise younger staff members and see the effects of that advice, even as I continue to work with Drexel Burnham's top management.

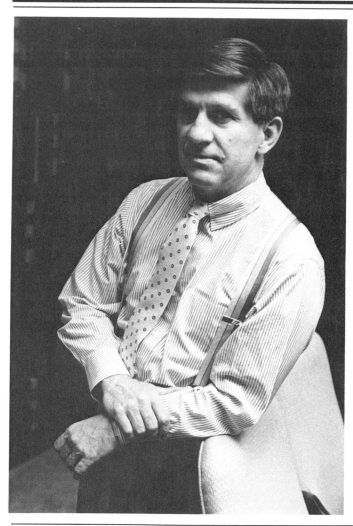

G. Chris Andersen
executive

Managing director of Drexel Burnham Lambert Incorporated, Chris is wearing one striking combination of his trademark items—color and pattern coordinated tie and suspenders. Here he carefully chooses three patterns of different sizes and varying scales: a yellow-and-blue-spaced foulard tie and wide-striped pastel suspenders on a closely striped blue tab-collar shirt.

Fred Joseph is CEO. He told me, "Since you spoke to us at DBL, I find our people dress with more confidence, which reflects itself in their appearance and presence."

Also at Drexel Burnham, managing director G. Chris Andersen has a uniquely different viewpoint. "I did some theater work in college and discovered how crucial to a role it is to be in correct costume. Dress rehearsal was far more exciting than regular rehearsals. When I get up each morning I review my calendar and see what role I'll be playing. I make sure that my costume is appropriate for that role."

When I take my seminars to the West Coast, I always make a point of dropping in to see Michael D. Brown, managing director at Drexel Burnham's Beverly Hills operation. Recently Mike told me, "In my case, I've always been interested in dress. But with your help, I have a much heightened awareness. I pay more attention now and notice how others are dressed.

"In fact, I even button my suit coats now. I had always been rather casual and never buttoned them before. Now that I realize how important these small points of grooming are, I can see how much better they make a man look."

Dr. Richard Cyert is president of Carnegie-Mellon University, in Pittsburgh, Pennsylvania. He began our conversation by recalling, "It is part of the academic cult to downplay clothes. As I moved into an executive position and saw others at that level, however, I began to like their finished, groomed look. I got more interested in clothes, particularly in buying clothes that fit me better.

"European shirts fit better than those made in America," he said. "They are trimmer. The French, in particular, make shirts with a better fit. The thing I dislike most about American-made shirts is their tendency to blouse. I used to like button-down collars. Now I think the perfect shirt is one with French cuffs, a straight, slightly short collar, and lightly starched."

Dr. Cyert was wearing a tiepin. "I like pins like this opal one I'm wearing, the kind that go through the tie. I guess you could say that tie tacks are a trademark of mine.

"I also like cuff links. One of my favorite pairs has the crest of Gonville and Caius, one of the colleges of Cambridge University in

England, where I used to teach. They were a gift. I also have some that used to be my father's which have his initials on them.

"Ties point up some of the mistakes I notice; not many men are interested enough in color. Somehow, particularly in past years, they felt that it wasn't masculine to be interested. That's certainly changing. You want to look your best. But most men need help."

A designer who is at the very center of the clothing industry, Andrew Fezza is noted for his relaxed, unstriving sportswear and weekend components. I questioned him about the relationship between casual clothing and traditional office wear. He sees no conflict. He feels that conservative men are starting to pay much more attention to the clothes they wear away from the office.

"Men who dress traditionally at work," he said, "want to dress in a relaxed manner on their own time."

Mr. Fezza sees traditional clothes being mixed with some of his unique sweaters and pleated pants—during nonbusiness hours, he stressed—to create what he calls a "fun wardrobe" for casual wear.

He sees nothing wrong with a businessman's clothes attracting a slight amount of attention. "Someone who makes an effort and has given some extra thought to how he dresses gains more recognition. He is regarded as an individual."

Robert Green is currently president of McRand Corporation, in Lake Forest, Illinois. I asked him to comment on whether he had noticed any changes in his managers' appearance and manner following a workshop I had conducted at J I Case, the construction and farm equipment manufacturer, a few years ago during his tenure there.

"There was a real difference: better coordination, both in color and materials. Sportscoats were a big thing with a lot of these people. They didn't wear the traditional three-piece suit, but they did wear a sportscoat, shirt, and tie. They still do—but you showed them how to coordinate them.

"I remember the green suits and the brown ones some used to wear before they attended your workshop. Also, at store managers' meetings, we used to see some hideous ties—ones that looked like you'd stirred up a fruit salad—worn with hound's-tooth sportcoats. All of a sudden those things started disappearing. And the improvement had an effect on the people who worked for the managers. It carried down to a lot of the staff. The managers cleaned up their acts and the rest followed. The image changed."

Paul H. Pearson, president of Security Mutual Life Insurance of New York, made several brief and to-the-point comments in response to my inquiry.

Paul H. Pearson
executive

"Good grooming—like good judgment—is something that gets noticed most when it is conspicuously absent," comments flawlessly groomed Paul Pearson, president of Security Mutual Life Insurance Company of New York. Sharp color contrasts and a perfect haircut contribute to a well-groomed look: A dark wool suit and carefully knotted tie sharply contrast his white shirt.

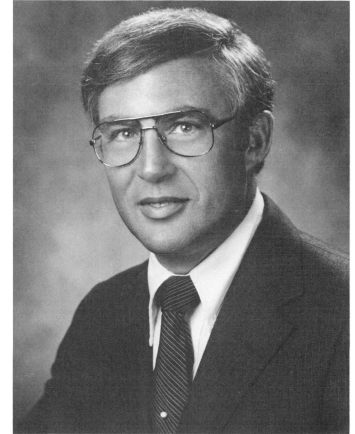

"The best total fashion statement the well-groomed executive can make may be none at all.

"Personal grooming and clothing styles of top management should be consistent with the public image their corporation chooses to project. It should be an image of self-discipline—looking and feeling your best to give your best.

"Good grooming, like good judgment, is something that gets noticed when it is conspicuously absent."

Stanley Marcus, a Texan and a maverick, built a family business into the immensely successful network of Neiman-Marcus department stores. He is a man of many opinions, always stated tersely and wittily. When we talked, he shared these Marcusisms:

"In the real world, a great man will overcome any superficiality of appearance, any deficiencies of dress. But executives on the rise may be judged by their dress more than those who have already reached the top.

"Men, like women, have started using clothes as prestige signals. Today wearing an Hermès tie automatically stamps them as $50 tie men, just as wearing a Countess Mara tie twenty years ago stamped them as $25 tie men. Presumably by the year 2,000 there will be another tie that will stamp one as a $100 tie man. For a while, status had men wearing Gucci loafers. But they fit so badly that a lot of men decided to go for comfort."

John Silton, managing partner of the accounting firm of Coopers & Lybrand in Washington, D.C., commented on the importance of an executive's clothes:

"If you look like a slob and you're a genius, you can get away with it. But in our company we have as part of our evaluation system—for people at the partners' level—a category we refer to as executive presence. It refers to an individual's leadership quality, his sense of self-confidence. Some people walk into the room and everyone notices them; others sort of blend into the wallpaper. A person's appearance heavily influences his executive presence evaluation.

"How much does the way he dresses tell you about a man? It indicates his level of self-respect and his taste. We assume that good taste

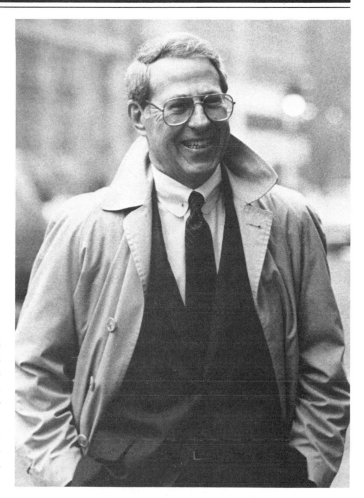

John F. Silton
executive

An upturned collar on his open
  single-breasted tan raincoat
  and his casual stance reflect the
  relaxed personality of Coopers
  & Lybrand's managing partner
  in Washington, D.C. On Silton:
  a charcoal gray wool suit, burgundy silk tie, white club collar
  cotton shirt with eyelet collar
  bar.

in clothes goes with good taste in other things. Of course, I've seen some
well-dressed, absolutely boring people. But that's life, and to be expected.

"Shoes are probably the biggest problem in terms of mistakes I've
noticed in other executives. They buy new suits, but not new shoes. And
they don't shine them often enough."

When I asked Mr. Silton if executive presence and good taste are
communicable, he said, "After you spoke to our partners, I saw a new
awareness. People talked about your program. And in the past few years
it has been reflected in their dress."

I asked Joseph J. Guiffre, senior vice-president of Metropolitan Life Insurance Company, what he learns from the way a man dresses.

"It tells me a lot. It tells me whether it is a customary thing for him to dress that way or if he's just doing it to *impress* me momentarily. Does he feel comfortable in what he's wearing? His clothes don't have to be expensive, but they should fit well and be in good taste. *It doesn't have to be my taste.* He should wear what flatters him. It can be more stylish than my clothes, but not so avant-garde that it's in the next century.

"Men should have some individuality in their dress, but not for shock value, or merely because they're trying to impress. Sometimes, if they dress outlandishly, I think it's because they're insecure or trying to get attention. Often how they dress tells how confident they are."

Recently I was asked to give several workshops on a Mediterranean cruise offered by the distinguished Royal Cruise Line. The chairman and owner of the line, Pericles S. Panagopoulos, was intrigued by the fact that I was writing a book on men's dress, and agreed to contribute his thoughts on what clothes say about a man and how he can dress to express confidence and personal style:

"No matter what they say, people attach tremendous importance to how a person looks. A clean, sober, and fashionable—without being exaggerated—appearance attracts attention and disposes people to see us in a positive way. By 'fashionable without being exaggerated,' I mean that a man's suit should not be a fancy one, but he has the option of wearing fashionable accessories such as shirts, ties, shoes, belts—maybe even a waistcoat. Ties in particular are an easy way for a man to follow the trends of time."

Donald M. Fordyce, chairman of the board and CEO of the Manhattan Life Insurance Company, a division of Manhattan National Corporation, has a right-to-the-point approach to dressing for excellence.

"I am always in pursuit of excellence, and in that pursuit, I believe appearance is critical. I believe the key to appearance is how much taste, or lack thereof, one reveals in the clothes he wears. The amount of money one spends on clothes does not ensure taste. Taste comes with a good

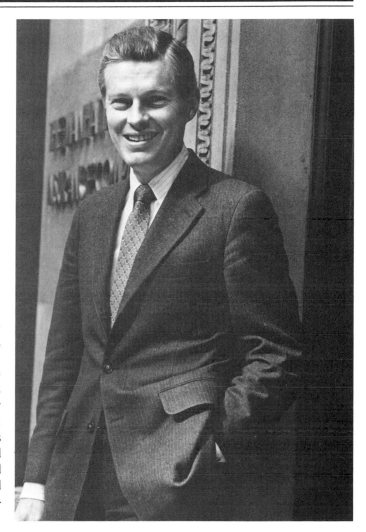

Donald M. Fordyce
executive

The chairman and CEO of Manhattan National Corporation, a financial services company, Donald Fordyce dresses traditionally. He wears only Hermès ties and accomplishes easily what many regard as difficult: He coordinates three patterns and achieves an integrated look. Notice the pin-striped gray wool suit, close-patterned silk tie, and spaced-stripe cotton shirt with French cuffs.

understanding of color and the match of each piece in the ensemble. This understanding has to evolve through continuous awareness and, possibly, with the assistance of a professional."

Donald Fordyce feels so strongly about encouraging an appreciation of excellence in dress in those around him that for three consecutive years he has given dress-oriented holiday gifts to the six members of his Operating Committee. The first year each received an Hermès tie; the following year they got navy blue cashmere blazers from Paul Stuart; and on the third Christmas their gift was a camel-hair blazer and charcoal gray slacks, also from Paul Stuart.

The Lilliston Corporation of Albany, Georgia, is a significant presence in the farm equipment industry. James C. Mainwood, president, wears a sportscoat—a strikingly handsome, well-fitted, and expensive one—to the office more often than not. He shared his views on dressing for business:

"There's no question that good taste helps open the door. It makes the presentation and it sticks with a lot of people. It tells you that people have an interest in themselves: that they have *pride* in themselves.

Daniel Berg, president of Rensselaer Polytechnic Institute in Troy, New York, has had a brilliant career both in industry and in university life.

"Working with industrial companies as a board member has caused me to accommodate my style to that environment. I have changed my style, but I have not compromised what I consider to be my standards. One does dress differently for different audiences so as to be comfortable, not out of place, and to feel well dressed. When I was in industry I had many suits from a Hong Kong tailor that were made with a more English styling. When I left Pittsburgh to go to RPI, that style of dress seemed out of place. Although the clothes were well made, they did not agree with the new environment and that encouraged me to make another stylistic change.

"Everything a person decides upon and uses says something about that person. The car he drives, the movies he goes to, the music he listens to, and the newspapers he reads—all tell you something. Clothes tell you immediately, of course, because one sees them right away. The signals can be misleading; but since the style and type of clothes are determined by the individual wearing them (no one is twisting his arm to wear any particular style), they can be revealing—often, I believe, accurately so."

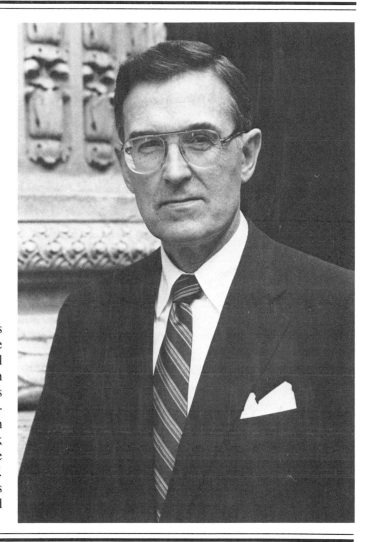

Daniel Berg
educator

Dan Berg's mode of dress brings
the corporate boardroom (he
has been a director of several
companies) to the campus in
Troy, New York, where he is
president of Rensselaer Polytechnic Institute. He wears an
updated American-cut dark
blue suit, striped silk tie, white
shirt, and white handkerchief.
No flourishes or frills—Berg is
direct, straightforward, and
convincing.

Finally, to bring my search full circle, I talked to a man who is
president of an influential organization, an educator, and a leading figure
in the world of style and clothing. Marvin Feldman, president of Fashion
Institute of Technology (F.I.T.), told me: "I have found that good clothes
are available only at a few stores. Of course, the cut and quality of those
clothes say quite a bit about the man who wears them. Recently I

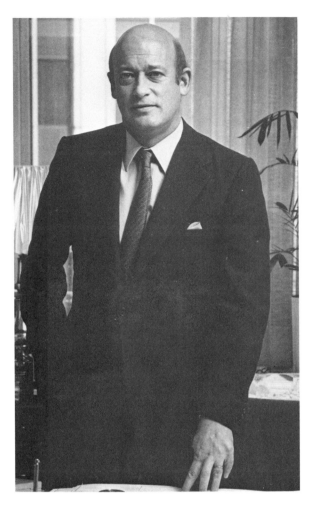

Robert A. Meister
executive

Robert Meister's clothes are custom-made by Europe's finest tailors. Details include an ice blue spread-collar shirt, fine silk tie, pocket square—nothing very tricky, but very well-made. He is vice-chairman of the board and director of the insurance firm Fred S. James & Company of New York, Inc.

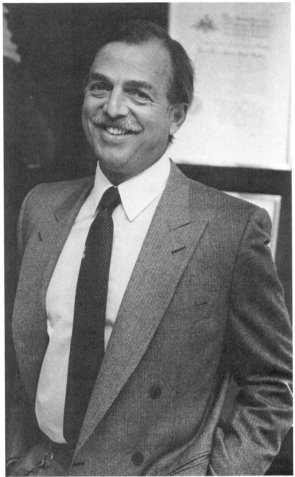

Allan R. Tessler
attorney

Tessler's cosmopolitan appearance is precisely right for a senior partner in the powerful and prestigious firm of Shea & Gould. His clients include some of the more celebrated names on both sides of the Atlantic. Here his dapper medium gray double-breasted wool suit, fashion-forward shirt with slightly shorter point collar, pindot silk tie, gold pocket watch, and well-trimmed mustache all contribute to a non-threatening "facilitator" approach and an air of individuality.

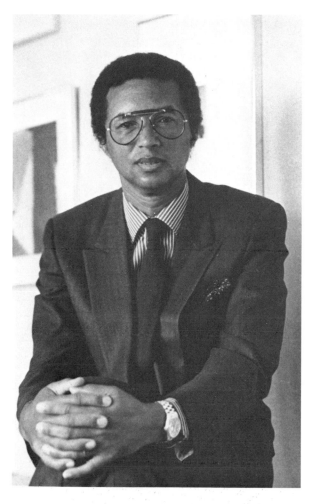

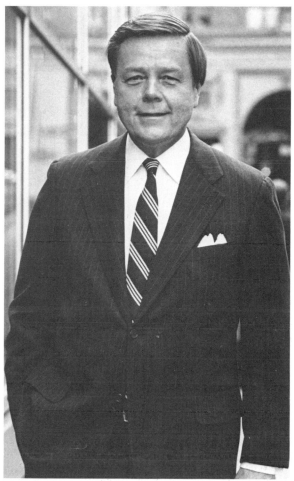

Arthur R. Ashe, Jr.
athlete, entrepreneur

John J. Schornack
executive

Photographed in the library of his Manhattan home, Ashe shows the composure and control that attracted world acclaim at Wimbledon and Forest Hills. Confidence and a sense of individuality allow him to carry off an uncommonly bold striped shirt. A large-scaled dress watch is his most visible accessory.

As vice-chairman of Arthur Young & Company, John Schornack dresses in the crisp yet subdued manner appropriate to the leader of a Big Eight accounting firm: well-tailored midnight blue wool suit, white cotton point-collar shirt and linen handkerchief, navy-and-white-striped repp silk tie.

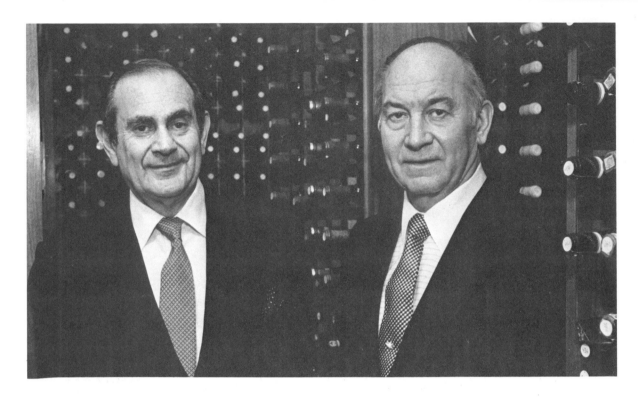

Tom Margittai and Paul Kovi
restaurateurs

Facing the camera in the wine cellar of their world famous restaurant, The Four Seasons, are owners Tom Margittai *(left)* and Paul Kovi. They make it a point to wear sophisticated business dress. Margittai is in a wool double-breasted suit, spread-collar shirt, small-patterned silk pocket square, and "neat" patterned silk tie. Kovi coordinates a woven silk tie and a white contrast collar on an unusual horizontally striped shirt. The two men are "on" day and night and unfailingly dress the part.

Kenneth C. Nichols   FACING PAGE, TOP
executive

His dark tie, eyeglasses, and vested gray suit offer a well-chosen contrast to his white shirt and silver hair. Ken Nichols is president of Home Life Insurance Company.

William R. Dill   FACING PAGE, BOTTOM
educator

President of Babson College in Wellesley, Massachusetts, Dill retains an unmistakable New England aura. His choices: natural-shouldered gray-blue shadow plaid suit, cotton broadcloth point-collar shirt, and silk school tie. "In dress, a college president's options can range from Walden to Wall Street. My preferences are for the conservative."

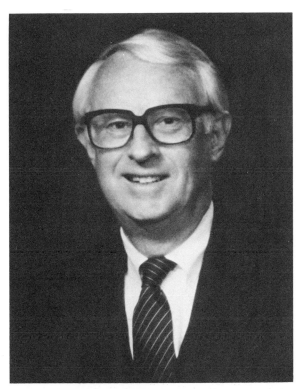

Kevin Harrington
assistant district attorney

BELOW

On the steps of the New York State Supreme Court in his yellow "power" tie, Harrington says, "When dressing for court, your clothes should send a message to a judge and jury that you are your own person, but one who plays by the rules." The well-cared-for leather briefcase and polished lace-up shoes show he plays by the rules. His natural hairstyle and his suit's slim silhouette add a dash of nonconformity.

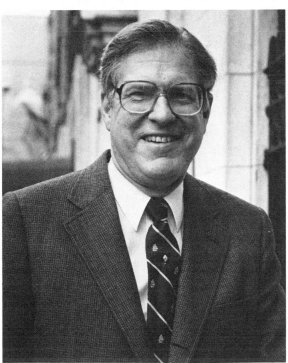

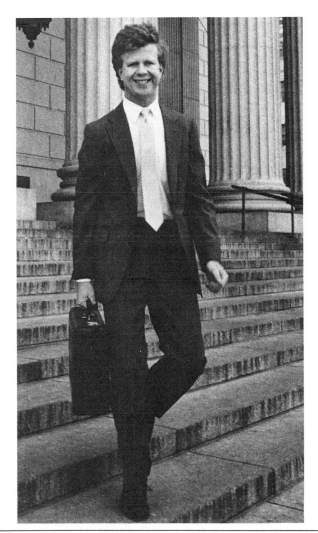

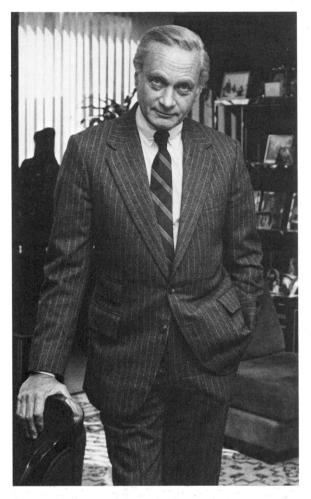

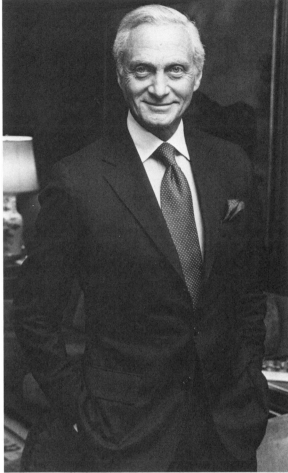

Morton A. Kornreich
executive

Although an identical twin, the chairman of the Kornreich Organization, insurance services, achieves an individual look through subtle details—a collar bar, perfectly groomed hair, an impeccably tailored gray shadow-striped suit with small ticket pocket.

Matthew R. Kornreich
executive

President of the company he co-heads with his twin brother, Matthew Kornreich says, "We shop separately but often are amazed to find that we have selected the same item—maybe even in the same color." His choices emphasize the traditional over the trendy: wool single-breasted three-button suit, spread-collar cotton shirt, paisley pocket square, and small-patterned jacquard silk tie in a half-Windsor knot.

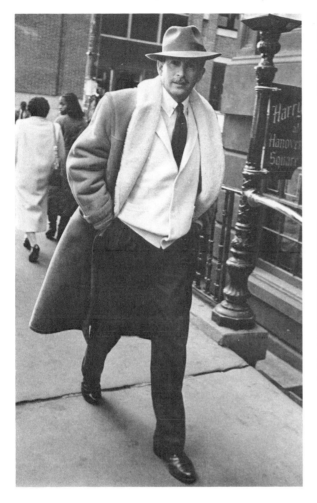

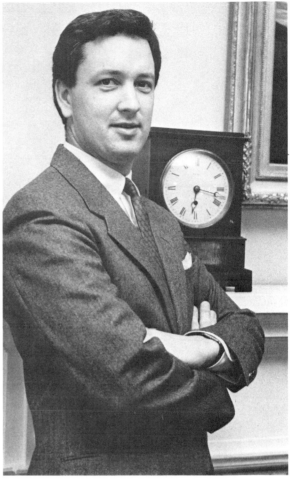

Roger Baugh
men's clothing designer

Baugh, winner of the Cutty Sark Menswear Award, 1986, combines casual yet dressy elements—fedora, full-length double-breasted shearling coat, pleated trousers, and lapeled cardigan. The designer wears neutral colors that repeat—and flatter—his fair coloring.

Brian Stewart
social New Yorker

Brian Stewart's noted taste in artwork and antiques extends to his choice of clothes: cashmere herringbone-weave suit, pinpoint oxford cloth button-down shirt, silk Hermès tie, white linen handkerchief, and a slim Le Coultre gold watch—a family heirloom—just visible under his shirt cuff.

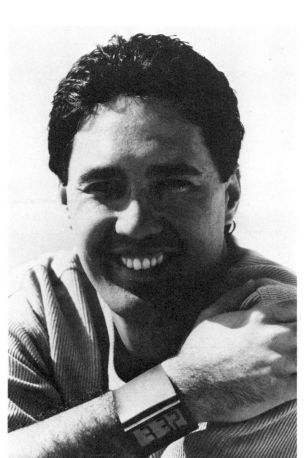

Eugene A. Cernan
astronaut

BELOW

Captain Eugene Cernan, the only man to have gone to the moon twice, has the distinction of being the last man to leave his footprints on the surface of the moon. He is now president of the Cernan Corporation, a consulting firm in the commercial space industry. Here, complementing his striking white hair, he wears a wool two-toned striped suit, silk foulard tie, and white button-down shirt.

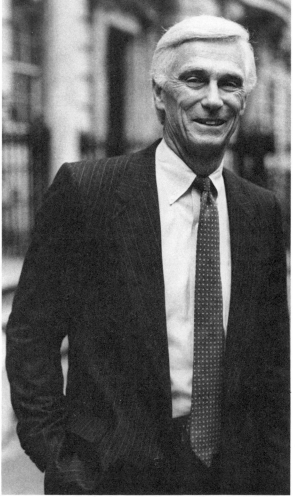

Ron Darling
pitcher, New York Mets

ABOVE

Making his best pitch for both the Mets and the Youth Drug Prevention Campaign of New York State, Ron Darling has the youth and self-confidence to wear a strikingly overscaled sports watch. In casual clothes or pin stripes, Ron Darling is the one to beat.

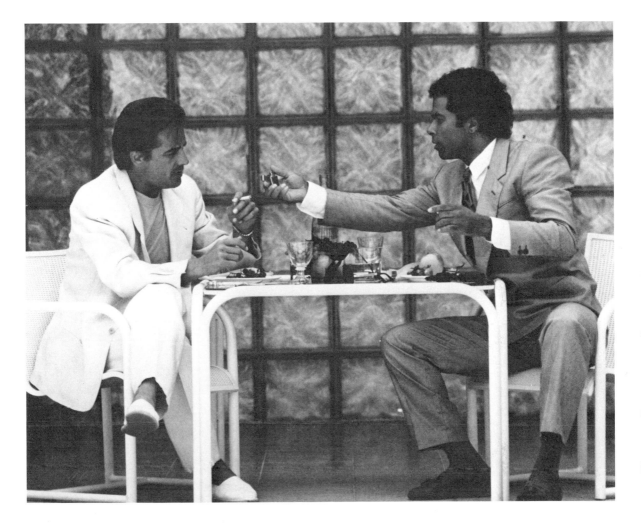

Don Johnson and Philip Michael Thomas
actors

Don Johnson *(left)* and Philip Michael Thomas, stars of TV's hugely successful show "Miami Vice," are dressed casually, but their clothes are top quality: Note the open vent on the sleeves of Johnson's linen blazer and on Thomas's double-breasted cotton suit. Both looks are perfect for weekend or resort dressing. The necktie works here but would be too flamboyant for business situations.

attended a Board of Directors meeting. Every man wore a gray suit; all the suits were good, but two were superb. Those men stood out.

"I wear a tie suitable for each occasion. Generally my clothes are very traditional except for the tie. The F.I.T. tie is a solid navy blue silk tie with a subtle F.I.T. pattern. When I am making a plea to the state legislature on F.I.T.'s behalf, I wear my F.I.T. tie. At other times I might wear the State University tie. On St. Patrick's Day I wear a green tie.

"As to mistakes I commonly see others making: mixtures and contrasts of different fabrics and textures that don't go together."

Each of these ultrasuccessful men acknowledges the importance of excellence in dress. They have, I hope, helped convince you of the advantages you will start to gain almost immediately when you upgrade your image. So we'll begin the process at once in the next chapter by taking stock of *your* own wardrobe, *your* interests, and *your* needs. And you will begin to make dressing well part of your reach toward excellence.

3

Building a Core Wardrobe

Right here, we're going to start talking about *you*. While the advantages of dressing for excellence apply to everyone who is in business, there are variations in applying those principles. Your preferences, your accommodations to your particular needs, and your life-style are only a few of the many factors that combine to form your personal style.

Have you ever sat down and asked yourself questions, analyzed the answers, and come up with a definition of your own style?

To give you a base for getting the most out of the tips and hints and formulas that fill this book, you will want to take stock of where you are in your career, what kind of work you do, the nature of your social life, and what you are really like—and convert that knowledge into a confidence- and admiration-assuring future.

So answer yes or no to each item in "The Dress for Excellence Questionnaire."

YOUR LIFE AT WORK

Yes No

1. ☐ ☐ Are you concerned about whether it is wise to dress better than your clients or customers? (See chapter 20.)

2. ☐ ☐ Do you know how to select clothes that play down your worst features and emphasize your best points? (See chapters 4, 9.)

3. ☐ ☐ Is much of your business conducted at lunches, dinners, or other nonoffice sites? (See chapters 17, 18.)

4. ☐ ☐ Does your office offer opportunities for variety—that is, times when a suit is essential, times when a blazer is fine— and do you know just when to wear which? (See chapter 20.)

5. ☐ ☐ If you are invited to the company's top producers' conference at a resort, do you know the right clothes to wear? (See chapters 17, 19.)

6. ☐ ☐ With a gray suit, certain kinds of shirt and tie combinations are entirely wrong. Any doubts about which they are? (See chapters 8, 9.)

7. ☐ ☐ Do you make presentations before groups of more than five or six? (See chapter 10.)

8. ☐ ☐ Do you know how to dress to win attention and admiration from women? (See chapter 16.)

9. ☐ ☐ Several types of ties are inadmissible to the business world. Do you know which they are? (See chapters 8, 9, 10.)

YOUR SOCIAL LIFE

Yes No

10. ☐ ☐ Does your position allow you to dress casually, even flamboyantly, in social situations? (See chapters 17, 18.)

Yes No

11. ☐ ☐ Are you sure of how to dress for business, but not always certain of what to wear for evening and weekend social occasions? (See chapters 17, 18.)

12. ☐ ☐ If visiting Dallas, Connecticut, or Minneapolis, are you confident that you'll wear the right clothes when your host says, "The evening will be casual"? (See chapter 14.)

13. ☐ ☐ Some colors emphasize your best features. Are you wearing the ones that flatter you? (See chapters 4, 9.)

14. ☐ ☐ Do you look better a few days after a haircut? That is, does the barber sometimes leave you with a "shorn sheep" appearance? (See chapter 15.)

YOUR TRAVEL and CLIMATE ACCOMMODATIONS

Yes No

15. ☐ ☐ Do you travel frequently on business? (See chapter 14.)

16. ☐ ☐ Would you like to know how to avoid a suitcase full of wrinkled clothes? (See chapter 14.)

17. ☐ ☐ If you were going to New Orleans or Los Angeles, would you know whether to wear summer or winter clothes? (See chapter 14.)

18. ☐ ☐ Do you know how to dress between seasons in what is called "transitional dressing"? (In autumn, on occasional warm days; in spring, when there's an unexpected nip in the air.) (See chapter 20.)

19. ☐ ☐ Do you know the trick of using light-colored wools and gabardines or dark-toned cottons to help span the seasons? (See chapter 20.)

20. ☐ ☐ Do you know how to travel with one suit and make it look like four different outfits? (See chapter 9.)

YOU IN THE WORLD OF CLOTHING

Yes No

21. ☐ ☐ Any doubt about such matters as how wide the correct lapels are this year? And what width tie goes with them? (See chapter 8.)

22. ☐ ☐ Wearing two patterns at once calls for knowledge, flair,

Yes No

and confidence. Are you reluctant to try it? (See chapter 10.)

23. ☐ ☐ Clothing store tailors sometimes exert too heavy an influence on customers. Do they determine, to a large degree, the style and fit of your suits? (See chapter 6.)

24. ☐ ☐ Are you puzzled about how experts judge quality in the construction of suits and shirts? (See chapters 6, 8.)

25. ☐ ☐ If you are one of the 9 percent of the total male population who is color-blind, do you know how to dress well even though you can't distinguish between certain shades? (See chapter 9.)

26. ☐ ☐ Are you aware of the "messages" these suit styles convey when you wear them: natural shoulder, padded shoulder; single vent, double vent, no vent; single-breasted, double-breasted? (See chapter 6.)

27. ☐ ☐ Do you know the three colors that are appropriate for business suits? (And the five shirt colors that are worn by top businessmen?) (See chapters 4, 8, 9.)

HOW MUCH ARE YOU WILLING TO SPEND?

Yes No

28. ☐ ☐ Do you regularly spend $400 or more for suits? (See chapter 5.)

29. ☐ ☐ For most of your shirts, do you spend $30 or more? (See chapter 8.)

30. ☐ ☐ For most of your ties, do you spend $25 or more? (See chapter 8.)

31. ☐ ☐ What is the ceiling amount you would spend for a suit? $_____ A shirt? $_____ A tie? $_____ A pair of shoes? $_____.

Your Life at Work. Questions 3 and 7 help you establish the demands and characteristics of your work. They are part of your corporate profile. But all the others refer to *you.* If you answered yes to 1 and 6 and no to 2, 4, 5, 8, and 9, you realize that you can use some help. That's great: Awareness is the first step to perfection.

You are in the same boat as hundreds of managers I have talked to in the last few years. The answers to your problems, and dozens of others, are right in the chapters I've indicated.

Your Social Life. Question 10 is a profile question. If you answered it no, you work in an exceedingly straitlaced atmosphere. Is it possible that you misinterpret what you regard as strictures? Is management really that concerned with after-office-hours affairs? If you answered yes to 11 and 14 and no to 12 and 13, your problems are not uncommon. Solutions are in the indicated chapters.

Travel and Climate Accommodations. Question 15 is another profile-establishing query. Nearly everyone answers yes to 16; packing is one of the more common vexations, and one of the easiest skills to learn. Questions 17, 18, 19, and 20, if answered no, are often-occurring problems that are laid to rest in the designated chapters.

You in the World of Clothing. If you answered no to questions 21 through 24 and yes to 25, 26, and 27, you are unusually sophisticated about clothes, from fabrics and designs through the retailing procedures.

Most businessmen are less knowledgeable. They answer yes to 21 through 24 and no to 25, 26, and 27. If you're in this second category, I promise you this: You can pass as an insider in well-dressed circles once you've absorbed the uncomplicated facts and formulas in this book.

How Much Are You Willing to Spend? If you answered no to the first three questions, you probably are not spending enough to create a truly first-class appearance. Question 31 extends your personal profile. If the amounts you've indicated are substantially less than the amounts in 28, 29, and 30, you won't find it easy to look your best. I'd say it is not impossible, but it is certainly difficult. The tips for astute shopping you'll find in every chapter will increase the odds in your favor.

You now have a fairly objective picture of where you stand on the road to appearance and style. As an immediate first step on that road I urge you to . . .

Green-Bag Your Closet

Several years ago I attended a presentation given by Robert Panté, the well-known West Coast authority on image. I was impressed by his concept of green-bagging your closet, and I would like to share his ideas with you here.

You know those large, superstrong green plastic bags that you use for collecting trash or autumn leaves? Get one, and let me look over your shoulder while you put it to a different use.

We're going to go through your closet and put in the bag all the clothes that have done you enough damage. Yes, I really mean *damage*. Although no one ever got a promotion just because he dressed brilliantly, all too many managers are passed over because they look wrong for the big new job. At work you constantly evaluate your equipment and supplies: Are they depreciated, worn out, or outdated? The same ruthless, discerning eye should be applied to your office clothes.

So reach in there and place in the bag:

Damaging group 1: Clothes that are in any way too small; jackets that bind in the elbows or armpits, or strain when buttoned; trousers that are short, tight, or put you at severe risk when stooping down; shirts that pinch or pull, socks that squeeze . . . even shoes that don't fit. Is there a hat that perches on top of your head like an afterthought? In the bag with all of them.

You may be in the minority whose misfitting clothes are too large. Maybe you are dieting, or your workouts have paid off. If the waistbands cannot be taken in and still look top-drawer, into the bag with them.

Am I suggesting that you get rid of wearable clothes and go out and buy new ones? Absolutely. Clothes that fit as I've just described are *not* wearable. Numerous charitable organizations in your community will be glad to accept the green bag's contents as tax-deductible contributions. You might try what I call "enlisting in the Salvation Army." Call the Army to come pick up the bag. Or send it to Goodwill Industries or any preferred religious group. But get them out of your closet.

Damaging group 2: Outmoded styles. Flared pants are an outstanding example. If you owned any, you probably got rid of them years ago. Yet sometimes we'll hold on to a hopelessly outdated piece of clothing, thinking that maybe it will come back into style. Or you figure, "I can always wear it on that weekend in the mountains."

Forget it. There's no good time for looking bad, just as there is no bad time for looking good. Shirts with long, pointed collars; sports jackets or blazers with dated lapels or slanted slash pockets; a sweater with ultrasuede trim; most of all, ties that are too wide, too narrow, or too shrill: There's room in the bag for all of them.

Damaging group 3: Just one more wearing. These are the clothes you love the most, the ones that have brought you compliments and admiring glances in the past: your favorite suit that's a little frayed at the shoe line (it's also losing a few threads at the right-hand pants pocket, and the lining has turned lacy under the arms).

"But I'll just wear it until it's ready for the cleaners and then I'll toss it out." You're stalling. You wear it once more, and once more—and another six months roll by. No more admiring glances, but you probably won't be aware of their absence. Those who see you, though, will be aware of something shabby about the way you look. They forget how fine you used to look. *Are things going wrong? Is he beginning to slip?* Without doubt, overage clothes send out strong "he's going downhill" signals. Clients or customers notice you're wearing four-inch collars. It has been years since stores were selling those relics. So observers conclude you can't afford new shirts.

You *can* afford new shirts and suits, but you can't afford a damaged reputation. Steel yourself, be tough about it—and break up your affair with those once-loved clothes.

Be conscious of *trading upward* every time you spend a clothing dollar. With some purchases, you'll be inching upward, a bit at a time. With others, you'll leap up to new compliment-arousing heights. Did your first purchase of a $30 tie send you home wracked with guilt? Possibly . . . but remember that every time you wore that tie you felt terrific.

Now you have clothes buying ahead of you. Be upbeat about it. It needn't be a chore, and it can give you a real lift. People who are wearied or frustrated by shopping don't realize they are frustrated by their own indecision and lack of confidence.

You may not believe it yet, but by the time you finish reading this book you will actually be looking forward to finding the right clothes and creating a new look for yourself.

I'm going to help you, step by step, know what's best for *you,* how to recognize it, and where to find it. We're going to build a wardrobe that gives you a total look of excellence. Instead of a random assortment of individual, fairly good components, you will have an integrated collection of the best in today's styles.

You will also have a sense of complete assurance in your looks that you may not have experienced before.

After you are comfortable with the basics of style (conferees at my seminars have called it "Basic Business, or Lois 1-2-3") you'll be ready to incorporate sophisticated special touches that give you the extra edge of personal style. That knowledge is in this book, too. When you reach that level, and are dressing with the style and flair that you have admired in others, you will have a wonderful sense of accomplishment.

My Five-Suit Formula

The first five suits in your new wardrobe should be selected in their order of importance. I believe you'd do well to follow this proven formula. It's one I use with many of my clients.

First suit: Solid dark blue. This one can be the natural-shouldered, Brooks Brothers look or the updated traditional American suit with only the slightest built-up soft shoulder and equally slight waist suppression. Everyone looks great in dark blue. A dark blue suit is the first choice of movers and shapers of commerce; leaf through *Time, Fortune,* a pile of annual reports, or the photographs in this book for confirmation.

Second suit: Dark gray, natural-shouldered or modified soft-shouldered.

Third suit: Medium gray with a subtle shadow or chalk stripe. Here, too, you have a choice of the natural-shouldered Brooks Brothers look or the traditional American, soft-shouldered cut.

Fourth suit: Navy blue with a subtle pinstripe or shadow stripe. My preference is the American-cut style over the Brooks Brothers, some-times called Ivy League or sack style. No matter what "they" told you in the placement department or in books you've read, the navy pinstripe should *not* be your first suit. It is the most formal daytime suit a man can wear and is just too dressy for many occasions. It is also more difficult to coordinate with shirts and ties than is a solid-color suit. A more subtle reason for waiting a bit to buy a navy pinstripe is that, of all the suits in your wardrobe, this one absolutely must be a good one. When it is anything less than fine, it looks tacky. Wait until you can afford a really good one.

Fifth suit. Here you have a choice among three different types. My preference is a summer tan suit, gabardine, or poplin. A second possibility is a lightweight gray. Third, a subtle glen plaid in medium blue or gray is a good choice, especially if your industry is a slightly relaxed one. Before you say you would never wear a plaid suit, be sure you know exactly what a *glen* plaid is (see chapter 10). A true glen plaid is a quiet pattern. In Europe fine tailors call the pattern Prince des Galles. Select one in colors that are muted and subtle; avoid any that are strident or demand attention. Be sure to give it the acid test for pattern match at seams, shoulders, and lapels (see chapter 6).

Five Suits . . . Plus

Although it is not precisely a suit, an important part of your core wardrobe is a navy blazer and a pair of medium gray or camel-colored slacks. (If you can afford it, a pair of each.) They are versatile, flattering, and practically a necessity.

How Far You've Come, Where You're Going

Think of the lift you've given yourself in the past half hour or so of reading this book. You have defined your appearance and personal style and have even begun to question how much you're willing to spend on dressing with style and flair. You've decided to toss out the marginally wearable clothes that have been holding you back. And you know the five-suit formula that has started other executives on their way to new levels of confident, powerful appearances.

Now you are ready to learn exactly how it's done. You will find all the facts you need about choosing, buying, altering, coordinating, and complementing your wardrobe in Part I, which follows.

PART I

THE
SECRET
OF THE
PERFECT
SUIT

4

How to Find a Suit That Makes You Look Like a Leader

Aperfect suit is like money in the bank. It is always there when you need it, always ready and always right. When you are unsure what to wear, it's the one you reach for, the one that works every time to give you an extra dose of self-confidence.

When you are dressing in the morning, you will spend time and give careful thought to what you will wear that day. But once having decided, you shouldn't have to think about clothes for the rest of the day. In the same way, buying a suit involves time and thought. But once you have it, the perfect suit is just that . . . perfect.

The CPW Philosophy

As you move your drive toward excellence into high gear, you may find yourself spending more dollars for clothing than you have been accustomed to paying. Sixty to 70 percent of that clothing investment will go for suits.

Price and value are interlocked. Compare the cost of an MBA from an Ivy League school with one from a local, community college—the worth of the costlier Ivy League degree is clear. Nor would anyone question the lasting values of a Rolls-Royce versus a Ford Escort. How are clothes any different?

Philip B. Miller, chairman of Marshall Field's, was quoted in a newspaper interview as saying, "Everyone wants value today, whether it's value at moderate prices or value at higher prices." It's interesting that Mr. Miller ignores even the possibility of value at bargain prices; with rare exception, it just doesn't exist.

Lasting values—suits that will be totally correct and wear-free in appearance five years from now—are what you are aiming for. In the pages that follow I'll tell you exactly how to make sure you are buying them, where and when to shop for them, what to look for, how to insist on the proper fit, and tips that even experienced shoppers may never have learned. Yet underlying it all is my cost per wearing, or CPW, philosophy:

A $375 classic navy suit that you could wear twice a week for three years comes to $1.20 a wearing: $1.20 for an image of confidence, control, and maturity all day long. A sale suit of greenish gray polyester, regularly $159 but catching your eye with a price tag of $80, projects an entirely different CPW formula. You wear it once, twice—and don't receive a single compliment. The third time you wear it, you begin to notice uneven seams; you have difficulty selecting a tie that's right (miracle ties just don't exist). On the morning of the fourth wearing you have a feeling you ought to wear something else, but you go through with it. There is a certain edge missing from your confidence all day. On the fifth day you go out to lunch and they seat you next to the kitchen. That day spent in the $80 bargain suit is the last. The suit goes into the green bag.

The cost per wearing of that suit, for five less-than-satisfactory excursions in greenish gray polyester, was $16—one of the most expensive "bargains" on record.

When I am asked, "What is a reasonable amount to spend on a suit?," I'm inclined to answer, "As much as you can reasonably afford." The idea is to "trade up" and spend more than you've ever spent before.

But the man who asked the question doesn't want maxims—he wants numbers. So I try to give him a range: $175 to $375 for a lightweight summer suit; $225 to $450 for a year-round weight; and for an especially fine suit, the crown jewel of his wardrobe, he might consider a $500 or $700 investment from one of America's finest manufacturers.

Those numbers can run a great deal higher. The world of bespoke (custom-made) tailoring extends well above the thousand-dollar mark. As for your own expenditures, I hope you will recognize the value of trading up, but you probably won't want to catapult all at once to the top price levels. Move up $100 or so every year or two and you'll be well on your way to the world of excellence.

Prices vary from store to store, city to city. If your fit is easy, or if you can wear nearly any model or cut of jacket because you are in great shape, you can expect to pay less for suits and still look good. If fitting you perfectly is a little trickier, the price may reflect it.

You'll know how to demand, and receive, a no-flaws fit after you read all the chapters here in Part I. A good fit can help a $250 suit look like one that costs $400 or $500 and will look that way for years.

What Looks Great on You?

Before you set out for a clothing store, where racks of suits are displayed for all shapes, sizes, and types, let's think for a few more moments exclusively about you. Do you know what looks great on you—not on the model in a magazine ad, but on *you*—when you walk into the office or are seated in a restaurant?

The style, the fabric, even the fit of the suit are universals. All should be perfect in a first-class suit bought at a first-class establishment. What renders your suit individually *you* is the effect that your *coloring* and your *shape* have on it.

The suit colors considered acceptable by the business world are limited to the three you've read about in my Five-Suit Formula: blue, gray, and on occasion, tan. The range of shades in each of these colors is huge. It is important to note that *business leaders choose blue and gray suits in the medium to dark range.* In the business world *brown suits are confined to light tan or a glen plaid in medium brown.* Right now I'm going to give you some basic rules concerning skin coloring and shades of suit fabrics, designed to narrow your choices to those tones that bring out the best in you. You'll then use shirts and ties for the lift and sparkle that well-coordinated colors invariably give a man's appearance. (There are whole chapters in Part II that detail precisely how to go about doing this.)

If you have dark hair, dark eyes, and sallow or olive coloring. Most gray suits are not flattering to you. Neither are most browns. Grays and browns are likely to have a "draining" effect, actually detracting from your natural good looks. That leaves blue.

Of course, you cannot build your entire wardrobe on blue. But you can emphasize it. If you are expanding your basic wardrobe to nine suits, you might want six blues. They should be well varied in pattern and tone. The fabrics could range from plain woolens and worsteds to mini-herringbones, stripes, and a classic glen plaid. Two dark or medium grays would suffice, but stay well away from the light end of the spectrum. And you could use one tan suit.

One cautionary note: Certain shirts you wear with your gray suits will flatter your skin more than others. A creamy shade of ivory (*not* the yellowish cast of beige), a crisp light blue, or a soft, clear pink—any of these will overcome the somber "gray look" that a man with your coloring can take on with a gray suit. *Contrast your dark coloring with clear colors in your suits and crisp or creamy colors in your shirts.*

If you have light hair and complexion or light eyes. With sandy hair and blue eyes, you look your best in a tan suit that repeats your hair color and a blue shirt that accents your eyes. You cannot, however, wear a tan suit all of the time. You are lucky because you have a *can't lose* choice: You can go either way. Wearing a tan suit during the warmer months is flattering because it repeats your coloring, yet the contrast offered by dark suits is also flattering. And, if you can manage a suntan, you increase your built-in advantage. The rule for men with light coloring is: *You look best by repeating your coloring.*

The flexibility enjoyed by men with light coloring extends beyond those with blond hair and light eyes. It includes blond men who are tanned and darker-haired men with light eyes. If you are in either of those categories, you can choose the color of your suit directly keyed to the occasion. You can wear almost any tone or pattern of blue, gray, or tan. Certain shades may be more flattering, or may be seen as authoritative and powerful (as explained in chapter 9). You may anticipate occasions when you will want to be seen as a facilitator—project a "let's work together" image. Softer and lighter shades of blue or gray convey that image and, with the right shirt and tie, they are exactly right for your skin and hair coloring.

For the man with gray hair, it is important to forget about the clothing combinations that looked so marvelous on you when your hair was brown. That was then. *Now gray is the color to repeat.* Regard gray in the same way that the man with sandy, red, or blond hair thinks of his light-colored hair—as an asset. You look great in all shades of gray. Muted tones, subtle mid-shade flannel, darker tick weaves or chalk stripes—the whole range of gray suits for the mature, confident executive will show you at your classic best. The new gray-stripe-on-white shirt, an understated bit of elegance, is a fine choice, too, but it needs a red or burgundy tie to warm up the chill gray tones. A pink or red-and-white-striped shirt is an excellent addition to a gray-haired man's wardrobe.

The varied range of black men's skin tones suggests a set of suit color choices that follow the same principles outlined for differing white skin tones. A rosy brown skin tone allows an unlimited choice of blue suits, from medium to navy, and tans/browns ranging from light camel through khaki up to medium brown. Yellow-beige and dark ebony skin tones are complemented by blues from the medium and darker segments of the spectrum. A white, ivory, or light blue shirt, particularly a stripe, allows a crisp maroon, blue, or multitoned tie to add a wonderfully attractive accent.

Oriental men look best in blue suits. Grays, from medium to mid-charcoal, are acceptable; but you do need that contrast of white, cream, light blue, or pink shirts. Avoid nearly every shade of brown and tan, even camels and khakis. They are "downers" on Oriental coloring and seem to fade into your skin color. The only relative of the brown family that you should invest in is a light beige or tan summer suit and a cream-colored shirt.

Suit Your Silhouette

Not the least of searching for a perfect suit is accommodating your own perception of your figure. It may not coincide with the world's view—you may be the only one in town who believes you are perilously thin, or a head too tall, or some such suspected deviation. But you believe it, and that's what we are concerned with.

Only when you are wearing clothes that offset the problem will you have the confidence and authority that should be yours. So search your hidden feelings: Do you secretly think you are too short, tall, thin, or heavy? For each condition, here are some general guidelines to consider before you set out to invest in a new wardrobe.

IF YOU ARE SHORT . . . Use vertical lines and details to draw people's eyes upward and give the illusion of greater height.

Suit features to look for:
- Pinstripes or chalk stripes (not too widely spaced) and other vertical patterns
- Jackets and blazers that are natural-shouldered and single-breasted, with narrow lapels and center vents
- Straight-leg trousers. Be sure they are not too short, and wear them with the slightest of breaks.

Suit fabrics to select:
- Light or medium weight
- Patterns or plaids should be small or medium size, never large or overscaled.
- Jackets and trousers should be of similar tones. When wearing gray slacks with a navy blazer, the slacks should be quite dark gray. A light/dark contrast between slacks and jacket will seem to cut you in half, making you look shorter.

Other garments:
- Long narrow ties; no bow ties
- Suspenders (if you feel comfortable wearing them)
- Shirt collars that have a narrow spread
- Bold, bright ties to accent your face

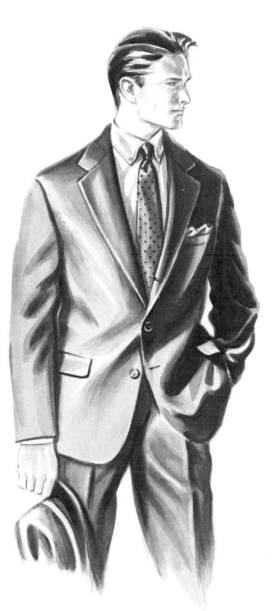 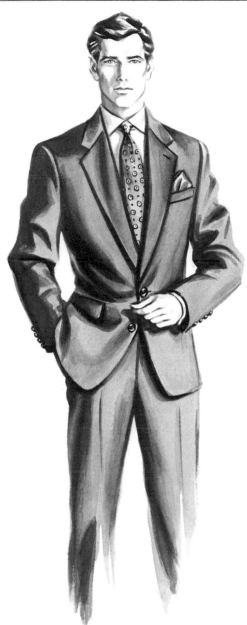

Traditional American cut, single-breasted, natural-shouldered "sack suit," often referred to as a Brooks Brothers cut (with button-down collar)

Updated traditional American cut, single-breasted and soft-shouldered (with spread collar)

IF YOU ARE VERY TALL . . . Use horizontal and diagonal lines and details, so that people looking at you will be moving their eyes across your figure rather than up and down, and will receive the illusion that you are shorter. In our society it is hard to imagine anyone unhappy because he is taller than average. But if you are in that minority, here are some neutralizing moves.

Suit features to look for:
- Horizontal lines and seams. Wear double-breasted suits with peaked lapels; on single-breasted models, choose slightly wider lapels.
- Cuffed trousers with a definite break
- Avoid pinstripes if you are tall *and* thin.

Suit fabrics to select:
- Medium to heavy weight, bulky textures
- Medium to larger size plaids or patterns; muted stripes
- If wearing a sportscoat or blazer, choose trousers of contrasting colors or tones. For casual wear, select bold, bright colors for either the upper or the lower half.

Other garments:
- Belt should be a shade slightly different from the color of the trousers, emphasizing the horizontal line.
- Shirt collars should have a slight spread. Avoid long, thin points.
- Choose slightly wider neckties with horizontal or diagonal patterns.
- For sportswear, opt for sweaters with horizontal stripes or argyle patterns.

IF YOU ARE THIN . . . You can wear stylish "layers" (sweaters, vests, two shirts) and easily create the illusion of width. Body portions that are very thin can be camouflaged. Try for lighter-colored suits within the acceptable ranges of blue, gray, and tan; dark colors tend to make you look thinner. (You realize, of course, that most people envy you. On the beach you may wish you were heavier; but in clothes you have the best of all "problems.")

Suit features to look for:
- Jackets and blazers with slightly wider lapels
- Double-breasted jackets with peaked lapels, perhaps with British-style double vents.
- Jackets with softly padded shoulders, slightly shaped sides
- Trousers with pleats
- Belted, straight-leg cuffed trousers
- If you are very thin, avoid pin-striped suits.

Suit fabrics to select:
- Bulky, textured—flannels or nubby tweeds, for example
- Glen plaids, mini-herringbones, and any other patterns appropriate for business
- When wearing a blazer or sportscoat, make use of colors. If you are tall, use sharply

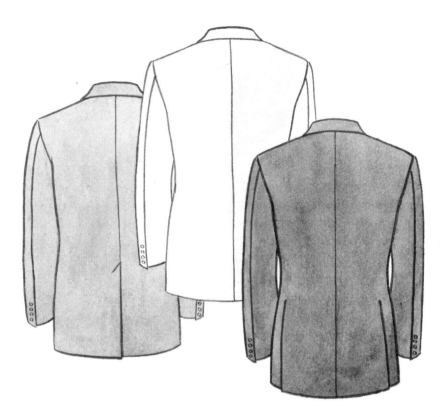

Vent types *(left to right):* traditional single vent; European no vent; double vent

contrasting jacket and pants—dark navy with light gray or tan pants, for example. If you are short, stay with dark navy blazer and dark gray pants.

Other garments:
- Shirt collars with slightly shorter points and a medium-wide spread
- For sportswear, striped polo and rugby shirts, sweaters with horizontal stripes or patterns

IF YOU ARE HEAVY . . . Focus interest and attention on your face by wearing compellingly interesting shirts and ties. Create an illusion of slimness by using vertical lines when possible. Dark colors in your suit can make you appear ten to fifteen pounds lighter.

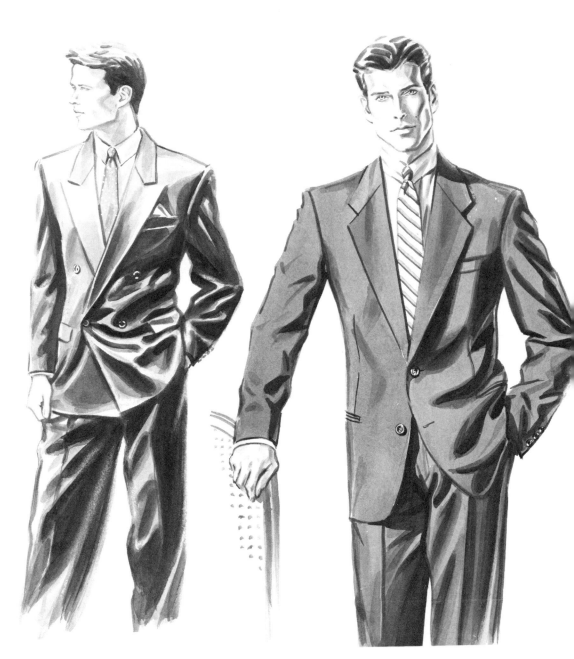

Double-breasted, peaked lapel
(with point collar)

European cut, single-breasted with
lightly padded shoulders (with tab collar)

Suit features to look for:
- Striped suits—pin, chalk, shadow—with closely spaced stripes
- Single-breasted suits and jackets
- Jackets with tailored (slightly padded) shoulders, straight sides, and center vents
- Straight-leg trousers. If you are wide in the seat (hips), avoid carrying anything in your back pockets.

Suit fabrics to select:
- Medium or light weights. Avoid bulky fabrics.
- Smooth textures
- Simple patterns. Avoid "busy" patterns, such as bold plaids, which add bulk visually.
- Cool, muted, and dark colors
- Blazers and trousers of nearly matching or similar tones

Other garments:
- Wear long neckties; avoid bow ties.
- Choose shirt collars that are low in back and on the sides, with a narrow spread. Wear button-down collars; avoid the horizontal lines of wide-spread collars.
- For sportswear, wear sweaters with vertical lines: light- or medium-weight cardigans; lightweight, vertically ribbed pullovers.
- Choose vertically striped dress and sport shirts.

IF YOU ARE UNEVENLY PROPORTIONED . . . You can achieve somewhat more balance by emphasizing the smaller of the unequal parts. **The rule is: Dark colors minimize; light colors emphasize.** A man with a broad chest and shoulders, slim hips and bottom, can gain proportion by wearing a dark blazer with contrasting trousers in light gray, camel, or winter white. Conversely, a man with a less developed upper body and broad bottom might wear a camel blazer with charcoal gray or navy trousers.

AN IMPORTANT OVERWORD. You can use many illusory tricks to create the look you want. You cannot eliminate all of the negative, but you certainly can learn to emphasize the positive. Knowing the simple secrets outlined above lets you show the world your best features. Nevertheless, it is essential to remember that while you are right to select clothes that are comfortable, feel good, and make you look your best, first things come first in the business world. If a style is flattering to you, but is not the accepted look of professionalism, you should opt for what is appropriate—for what is *serious* and excellent. As an example, suppose you are short. The books you have read and the tailor in the store tell you that cuffs on trousers are better left to tall men. But you know that all of the top men in your industry are currently wearing cuffs. Wear cuffs.

If you are a redhead and know that green is a flattering color for you on the golf course, don't elect to be the one guy at the office who comes to work in a green suit. It may flatter your face, but it will practically destroy your image. Do what works best for you within the framework of your stretch toward excellence.

5

The Right Time and Place to Buy a Suit

The Prime Time to Buy a Suit

Stores begin to receive and display their fall and winter merchandise in July and August. If you are looking for a fall/winter suit, I suggest that you schedule a visit to three or four likely stores at the end of August or during the first two weeks of September. By that time they will have received their new clothes for the season; they'll have a complete selection in all sizes. You will be far in advance of the late September surge of customers, which means salesmen will welcome you and be attentive.

As a customer, be aware of the trade-off implicit in the retailer's merchandising calendar. His stock and selection of sizes and models are at their fullest when summer turns to autumn. So, too, are his prices. Later, at the end of the season, he knows he is going to be left with unsold merchandise until he can start to move it again the following August. He'd rather mark it down heavily to move it out of the store and do what he can for his cash flow.

So you will find significant savings offered in early January sales—from 20 to 50 percent off on some of the original prices. Of course, you will be limited in your selection of colors and styles, and often there is a too-sparse representation in the popular size range, 40 to 42. On the other hand, you could find bargains waiting among the less common sizes. What one first-class store doesn't have, another may. If you have the patience, your savings might justify the time spent at the season's end.

The stock-and-sale cycle for lightweight suits is equally predictable. Stores' racks are full in early April and that's the best time to buy if you are prepared to pay full price. Markdowns of remaining summer stock traditionally begin on Fourth of July weekend. A lightweight suit bought then will still give you plenty of wear before the first frosts of October. So if you can postpone your buying until July, you will have that much more to invest in a suit—and enough left over to buy a few shirts to wear with it.

Where to Buy

It will be very much in your interest to buy a large percentage of your clothes in one store. The personnel will regard you, over the years, as a valued customer. You will know the manager, the salesmen, and—even more important—the fitter. But which store will it be?

To begin with the *won'ts:* It won't be an undiscovered gem of a place; a little boutique. The selection at such stores is too narrow and the styles too quirky for serious consideration. And it won't be a large department store that has a few high-end suits, but generally does business at the middle and lower ends of the quality scale.

If you live or shop in one of the larger cities, you may not be able to afford the very best store in town. But one at the next level will do just fine.

Make a list of four or five possibilities. Ask peers whose style you admire where they buy their clothes. Read newspaper advertisements. And look around: Check out a few of the well-known stores in your area.

Keep in mind that you don't want to begin an important relationship too far away. Immediacy is important for a quick drop-in when a tie or shirt is needed for an unexpected overnight trip. And nearness forestalls thinking of clothes shopping as a chore.

From among the candidates, select the store that rates highest in these essential qualities:

- **Several fine manufacturers' suits are stocked.** If the store uses its own label, ask the manager for the names of the makers. Two or more fine, traditionally reliable firms should be represented: Oxxford, Hickey-Freeman, Harry Lebow by Oakloom, Hart Schaffner & Marx, Cricketeer, and Southwick are among the better known ones. Famous designer names are less reliable for traditional business wear. You are concerned with business clothes, and most designer fashions are not classic enough for the business world.

- **A salesman whose taste and judgment are impeccable.** When you walk in, one salesman will approach you. In retailers' parlance the man who is "up" gets the next customer. But you are in no way obligated to follow the store's system of rotation.

  Unless you are immediately impressed with the salesman's manner and the way he is dressed, do not accept his offer to help you. "No thanks, I'm just looking," is what you say. Observe the other salespeople, and note the kind of customers they are serving. If you admire the look and style and manner of one salesman, wait until he is available. You approach *him,* and tuck his card into your wallet. Let him help you dress the way you want to look.

  That is all done the first time you shop in the store. After that, the ideal procedure is to phone ahead and make an appointment with your salesman.

- **An excellent tailor.** When I am asked how you judge a tailor's work before you've seen it, I confess it's easier to know if the light stays on in the refrigerator once the door is closed. But perfection is the only admissible level for your new suit's fit and alterations. If all else is right, and the first few moves by the fitter/tailor seem totally professional (details on this are provided in full in chapter 6), go with your inclination. Chances are, he won't disappoint you.

  But be tough. Insist on direct answers to any questions. Commit him to any changes you want made. There is still time to pull out—to take off the suit and say you've changed your mind.

If you do buy the suit, the first and second fittings can still be turning-away points. Anything that you feel unhappy about can and should be remedied. It doesn't happen often, and the store management may not be too cordial about it, but you should refuse to accept a suit that shows inferior or flawed tailoring. If the minuses outbalance the pluses, you should definitely visit another store the next time.

· **A store that tradition and experience tell you stands behind its merchandise.** Buy in any fine, well-established store and you will have no difficulty resolving problems. Even if it is a suit or pair of trousers you bought months ago, a first-rate store will accept a return or in some way arrange matters to your satisfaction. This holds true both for specialty stores—again, the better ones—and for department stores. (Specialty stores sell primarily clothing. Department stores sell large appliances and furniture as well as clothes.) Merchandise can be returned to a store for full credit by a charge account customer—no questions asked; no reasons need be given. If he is convinced that the merchandise is not up to the store's standard, the customer is the sole judge; he returns it and is not billed for it. Many demanding, perfectionist men have a policy of buying all their suits at stores where they have charge accounts so that returns are not a hassle.

Discount Stores: How to Know What You're Doing and What You're Getting

"What do you think I paid for this suit, Lois?" is a tricky question. It is often asked by an executive who comes over to me at break time during one of my seminars. Obviously he's confident his suit looks and fits like an expensive one, yet he may have bought it at a discount store for half its apparent value.

If, in fact, a suit picked off the rack at a discount store does look as classy as its wearer believes, several factors are at work: He has excellent taste, he spends a lot of time shopping, he is blessed with a flawless body, or he knows an excellent tailor.

I do know a few executives who buy their clothes in large barnlike discount stores at huge savings, and look as though they've been outfitted at Lord & Taylor or Brooks Brothers. *They can do it because:*

- They are careful. They examine each seam, pocket, and lapel for flaws. They know where to look and where imperfections might exist.
- They are knowledgeable. They understand what classic styling is, and they know what is trendy and soon to be passé. They recognize manufacturers' labels and are even familiar with identifying touches that tell them who made the clothes when labels have been removed. They have developed an eye by preshopping in the better stores.
- They ignore the store's personnel. They are their own salesmen, and they do have a brilliant tailor in his own little shop.
- They are willing to spend time.

I don't recommend your trying the discount route until you are fully confident of your knowledge about the clothing world. Also, time is money; for most businessmen, the return on their time doesn't make sense. But it is a misconception to believe that there must be something wrong with a suit that is sold for half price.

Yes, there are *seconds* and *irregulars*—flawed garments that don't meet manufacturers' quality control standards, and these may be unlabeled and unidentified. But in a reliable discount store, items that are seconds are usually marked as such. Often the terminology is "as is," but you must spot the particular imperfection for yourself.

However, not all merchandise offered at huge savings is imperfect. When people say, "You only get what you pay for," I say, "That's not *always* true." The owner of one of the East's most successful discount chains explains it this way:

"Suppose one of the big suit makers gets an order from Saks Fifth Avenue and Rich's in Atlanta. They each want 500 of a particular model. He makes 25 extra, for safety, and they're all first-run. No mistakes.

"Or he makes 2,000 and sells all but 60 to a couple of big stores. Those stores don't bother with small quantities.

"So the maker calls my buyer. He tells us what he's got, and what he'll take for the whole lot of 60. If he covers his cost, he's happy. We take out the label so no one gets embarrassed, put the suits on the racks, and move them out of here in three or four weeks. Our markup is small, and some lucky guy is wearing a $450 suit that he got for $229.50."

One thing I'm sure of: Anyone who is a dedicated shopper and knowledgeable enough to maintain his image in discount-purchased clothes spends more time scouting the right look in expensive stores than he does in actually buying the clothes at the discounter. It pays off for him, and is time well spent. But it's not for everyone, and maybe not at all for you.

What Fabric Are You Buying?

The quality and type of fabric from which your suit is made determine, to a large extent, its final cost. They also determine your satisfaction: Will the suit wear well and retain its shape and appearance for several years? To be sure of the answers to these important questions, let's take a quick look at the world of fabrics.

Wool, cotton, silk, and linen are called *natural fibers.* They are traditional, classic, and more expensive than the synthetics.

Wool's versatility and ability to be combined into so many weights, finishes, and textures makes it the most desired and most used fabric for men's suits and coats. In processing the raw animal hairs, yarn makers dye them, sometimes blending in synthetic fibers for added strength and wrinkle resistance. Cloth made of wool can be molded into shape, which is why tailors achieve such fine results when making coats and suits of wool.

Heavy-weight woolen clothes are among the warmest you can buy. Moths like wool, too. They are especially attracted to clothes that are soiled, and go directly to the stained areas of a garment. Unless you clean wool clothes before putting them away for the summer, moths may wipe out your investment in fine suits, coats, and sweaters right in your own closet. (Nothing looks worse than damaged clothes. These cannot be worn "just once more." They must be thrown out.)

Cotton is used in lightweight summer suits of poplin, seersucker, cord, tweed, and gabardine. Few suits or jackets are 100 percent cotton; customarily synthetics and wools are blended in to add weight, texture, form retention, and versatility. Yet cotton's qualities remain highly desirable. It is strong, lightweight, comfortable, and cool.

Cottons take dyes beautifully and are not subject to static electricity or to pilling (gathering of little balls or "pills" of fiber on the garment's surface). Cotton fabrics do wrinkle readily and tend to shrink if laundered rather than dry-cleaned, unless the yarn is treated chemically before weaving. Even when treated and dry-cleaned, they will shrink to a slight degree in the pressing.

Manufacturers make a big sales point of cotton summer suits' washability. My advice is to ignore that feature. You will be unhappy with the appearance of washed suits; they won't measure up to your requirements for excellence. You will always look slightly rumpled. Since you are going to send the suit to the dry cleaner, don't let the nonexistent economy of self-laundering influence your purchase.

Silk is to fabrics as gold is to metals. Kings and emperors wore it, and so did their queens. The most beautiful fabric I've ever seen is the patterned silk made in Venice in the 1920s by Fortuny, fashioned into gowns by the world's greatest couturiers—and still worn by the most elegant of the super-rich. Silk's incomparably smooth touch and texture is often blended with wool or linen into sports jackets for interesting texture and weight. Though high-style weekend wear often has silken components, pure silk suits are not worn by business leaders during office hours. "Too slick, too showy," is the consensus.

Linen, sometimes called flax, is an elegant and luxurious fabric. Its light weight and its tendency to carry heat away from the body make it a favorite cloth for summer-weight suits and jackets—expensive ones. Because linen fabrics wrinkle easily, manufactuers often produce them in a blend with cotton, silk, wool, or shape-retaining synthetics. Some manufacturers know that not everyone is familiar with the distinctive properties of linen. They sometimes put "Guaranteed to wrinkle" on the labels attached to the garment. Those who are knowledgeable about linen say it has "regal wrinkles." Ramie, a vegetable fiber grown in the Philippines, is relatively new to the clothing world. It has a linenlike look and feel, is less expensive than the real thing, and is generally used in combination with other yarns.

Linen adds luster and subtlety to a jacket or pair of trousers. There's nothing more rich, more perfect, than weekend outfits of ivory-toned linen. Yet I would never recommend linen for inclusion in your first round of clothes. Save linen and silk for expressions of confidence once you have the basics firmly under control.

Man-made fibers have been developed to add some specific qualities to natural fibers and sometimes to replace the natural materials entirely. But in terms of business suits, the use of man-made yarns should be restricted to blends with natural fibers. "Shiny synthetics" and "perfect polyesters" are *not* synonymous with quality.

The preferred blend is 55 percent polyester (more often than not it is Dacron, a registered trademark of the DuPont Corporation) and 45 percent wool. If you can find it, a little higher percentage of wool than polyester is preferable.

A blend needs little care. Its chief advantages are that it holds its press and is less expensive than pure wool. Another advantage is that certain stains are easier to remove from a blend than they are from all wool.

Today's look has moved away from the artificial perfection of the 1970s. Blow-dried and lacquered grooming, with every hair carefully in place, was the hallmark of the past decade's style. Today's look is natural: natural fibers, natural complexions, and tolerance for an all-too-natural wrinkle or two, particularly in leisure clothes.

Some men hate any sign of wrinkles. They don't care what the current thinking is on that subject. My own personal preference for the business world is for the "real" look of natural fibers. I find them more desirable than the unreal perfection of heavy doses of polyester. (I strongly believe that a man's shirt collar should be crisp and perfect, but a suit can have a few wrinkles.) Nevertheless, it is your choice. If you are uncomfortable with any sign of a wrinkle, you will probably be happier with a blended suit.

Suits worn by the most successful men are generally made of all wool. Occasionally they will supplement their wardrobes with a wool-polyester blend to avoid a rumpled appearance when traveling. You can find exceptions among the passengers in any elevator in any skyscraper. But I do want to emphasize the prominence of wool in the kind of wardrobe you will be building. Wool is traditional. It is rich in appearance and "hand" (a tailor's term for the feel of a fabric), and it is what leaders assume other leaders will be wearing.

Tightly woven wool fabrics are called *worsteds*. Among them are covert, gabardine, serge, and sharkskin. These hold their shape (and a crease) well. If you want all wool but hate wrinkles, stay with worsteds. Heavier, softer, more loosely textured finishes are called *woolens,* and include flannel, shetland, and tweed. Today's suiting fabrics of both types are customarily made of all wool or wool blended with polyester.

No need for technical explanations of how the weight of cloth is measured. Just keep in mind that heavy, winter-only suits are customarily made of cloth that weighs eleven or twelve ounces per square yard. You may find that weight too heavy and thus too warm, even in the coldest winter climates. Lighter year-round fabric, known as a "ten-month weight," is an eight-to-ten-ounce cloth; it is ideal for suits.

Do not make the mistake of thinking that because you live in a warm, humid climate, you cannot wear all-wool suits. The truth is that wool blended with synthetics is not nearly as comfortable as a very light, tropical-weight all-wool suit. All wool "breathes": The natural fibers allow air to pass through them. Blends containing synthetic fibers do not, which is why blends tend to make you perspire freely (they also retain perspiration odor). The better stores—the kind that you will be shopping in—carry a full selection of all-wool suits in all weights.

Of course, the weight of the wool fabric governs its suitability for year-round or warm-weather wear. But in every weight, "all wool" says all the right things about you.

6

How to Get a Perfect Fit

Your mission in the clothing store is clear and direct. You are there to buy suits that will allow other successful businessmen to recognize you as one of them. In those suits you will gain confidence. You will send out the message that you can be relied on for the highest responsibility.

A suit will do all this? Yes, if the suit is worn by a person who actually has those abilities. The point is, the suit will help you gain acceptance. It won't set up barriers. There will be no assumptions of "He doesn't seem quite up to it" to exclude you from having a shot at the top.

How to Look at a Suit

What are the touches that distinguish the best suit from a merely good one? When you are screening dozens of suits, looking for the better possibilities, exactly what are you searching for?

I asked Jack McDonald, president of Oxxford Clothes, Inc., to tell me why his firm's $750–$1,000 line is considered the best in the industry. He explained in detail, and I've summarized it as a set of criteria for selecting a suit, by whatever maker, of the highest quality you can afford.

When you examine an Oxxford suit, not all of Mr. McDonald's fine points can be discerned. But they are in there. Knowing them gives you an idea of what goes into a masterwork of garment making.

- The ingredients are the finest available. The wool is the best. The silk thread, the linings, the genuine water buffalo horn buttons—all are the very best.
- Each garment is cut *singly* by hand. More and wider seam outlets are left so that, when necessary, the clothes can be let out without losing balance.
- Stripes and plaids are matched perfectly at sleeve, shoulder, lapel, back seam, breast pocket, and pocket flaps, with no disruption to the pattern's line. This requires an extra one-quarter yard of material.
- The interfacing between the layers of the coat front, to give it body and shape, is canvas that has been cold-water-shrunk and specially dried. It is hand-basted to the coat, never mechanically fused. It always stays in place.
- The collar and lapels are hand-stitched to ensure softness and a perfect roll for the life of the garment. The collar contains approximately 1,350 stitches and there are 800 in each lapel.
- All edges are hand-stitched.
- Underarm shields are provided as protection against perspiration.
- Buttonholes are made by hand. They are worked on both sides of the opening—really two buttonholes one on top of the other—to prevent raveling.
- All buttons are sewn on by hand. The four buttons on each sleeve "kiss" one another in a precise arrangement.

- Pockets have a complete bellows on the inside, permitting the pocket to expand to the inside, rather than bulging to the outside.
- Trousers are constructed with a one-piece waistband in which the pockets are laid: smoother, thinner, and longer lasting.
- The fly lining is pleated down to prevent curling at the crotch.

Narrow Down the Salesman's Options

If you feel reasonably sure about the reputation of the store and the service you will receive, you might choose to be fitted for two suits during your first experience. But certainly you will want to see how they perform before committing any further. The safest course is to start by buying only one.

Two warnings are in order. Guard against the salesman's showing you anything today except business suits. No designer models, no sports jackets or blazers. You are there to buy a classic suit, either Ivy League or an updated traditional cut, with no special touches, no fancy stitches. All details should be classic.

Increasing numbers of under-forty managers, particularly in communications and glamour industries, are choosing a "fashion forward" look. Their suits are often without vents, are sometimes double-breasted and carry a designer label: Perry Ellis or Giorgio Armani or Ralph Lauren's Polo line. That's fine if you want to try it—later—maybe as a bit of weekend flair. But now, today, you require the *basics,* the traditional look of excellence.

And watch out for a rigid assumption, on your part or the salesman's, that your new suit must be the same size as your last one. Your shape changes over the years. More crucially, manufacturers' sizes vary, even from model to model.

Handling the Tailor

Is it worth $10 or $20 to help a $250 suit fit like a $500 one? That's hardly a question. And there's no question that the trick can be performed by the tailor who supervises your suit's alterations. (In a large specialty store or department store the fitter is your only contact with the tailoring staff. In that case the *fitter* is your man. In a smaller establishment the *head tailor* often doubles as the fitter. We'll use the terms interchangeably.)

Tipping the tailor is a wise investment. It is not considered gauche or demeaning. It is done all the time, and in the very best stores. Recently a man in my audience asked me how much to tip the tailor. My response: "Any amount from $5 to $20, depending on the extent of the alterations and how soon you need the work done. But any tip will make the tailor remember you."

It should be clear that this is an advance appreciation for the superb work you are going to receive. I remember the CEO of an Illinois bank, a rather short man who dressed superbly, telling me how he established a relationship in a Chicago store when he moved from San Francisco. "I told the manager I wanted the best fitter. I explained that I'm fussy, a little hard to fit, and sometimes have to come back for three fittings. I wanted to avoid that. He got the point. He knew it would run up his costs if they didn't make me happy; he made sure George took care of me. And I took care of George, right from the start."

Ask the fitter questions. Challenge him. Praise him and flatter him, and don't forget him at Christmas. Your appearance will reflect his gratitude.

The Fitter's Codes

The fitter's chalk marks on your suit are the tailor's guide for alterations. A single line means "reduce length or size." A line crossed by two slant marks means "expand."

And—slyest of all maneuvers—"R.C." written on the alteration ticket means "Remove chalk." That's when they figure you'll never know the difference.

Fit Is Forever

Be sure to have all necessary alterations done. Often a man buys clothes and thinks of the price on the ticket as the final cost. It's a price he's comfortable with, and he is unwilling to go beyond that figure. Most stores do simple alterations—the universal sleeve and trouser adjustments—free, but they charge for such work as raising collars or adjusting the seat. Do not decide that these corrections can be overlooked. Good tailoring and a fine fit are necessities, not luxuries.

It's true that women often can justify wearing their hems an inch or two long to save the cost of alterations. Their fashions vary every thirty-five seconds and no free alterations are available. But men do not wear their sleeves at the wrong length; they insist on perfection in that regard. Why overlook any of the other, equally important aspects of perfect fit? They are absolute requisites of dressing for excellence.

Trying It On: Eight Surefire Steps to Evaluate a Jacket's Fit

Your first move should be to try on the jacket of a top-quality dark blue suit in a eight-to-ten ounce fabric known as a "ten-month" suit. When you have found one that you think you like and are considering buying, put in its pockets all the items that you normally carry. The suit must fit as it will be worn in the world of reality, not as you see it in a clothing store. If you carry a wallet, an eyeglass case, and a datebook in your coat pockets, transfer them to the one you're trying on.

Make it absolutely clear to the salesman that you always return to the store for a *second fitting,* even though that may be stretching it a little. He ought to understand this at the start, and realize that anything less than perfection will be unacceptable. (Your reasons for asserting this, and what happens at the second fitting, will become apparent as you progress through this chapter.)

You are trying to determine the correct size and fit, so step up to the three-way mirror and look closely at these aspects of the jacket:

1. *Shoulders.* This is the first key to perfect fit. Any other part of the suit can be altered if necessary; the shoulders cannot. (No experienced tailor would attempt it. He knows that the line of the suit will be warped, no matter how skillfully he may restitch the seams.) If there is a bulge at the shoulder, or if it makes your upper arm muscle appear prominent, try another size or another model.

2. *Chest.* If the front of the jacket bulges or wrinkles at the lapel

area, it does not fit properly. It may be due to your body structure: a leaner or stronger development on one side. But before undertaking alterations to correct the problem, try another model or two. Ask the tailor if he can suggest a manufacturer who makes a suit cut on a pattern that is better for your body shape. You may find one that fits perfectly.

3. *Collar.* Here, using the three-way mirror is essential. At the sides and back the collar should be snug. It should not gap or fall away, and it must be no more than three quarters of an inch below the top of your shirt collar. Don't allow the fitter to drape the coat on you perfectly, right up snugly on your neck, and persuade you that the fit is correct. Be firm with him. Move around; button and unbutton the jacket; swing your arms; *then* see how the collar stands. Don't feel, however, that you cannot buy a suit that does not fit perfectly at the back of the collar. This is a minor adjustment for a good tailor. Ask him if he can alter it so it will be perfect and snug.

4. *Lapels* should lie flat. See that no ridges or bulges are caused by unevenness of the interfacing (the stiffening material between the layers of fabric).

5. *Armholes.* Occasionally suit buyers run into a problem after they have begun wearing a suit and conclude that it is too tight under the arms. Anticipate this by being absolutely sure that the jacket is full enough to ensure comfort. There should be no cramped feeling, no matter what position your arms may be in. (And remember, you have already placed in your pockets all the paraphernalia you usually carry.) Some of the more fashion-forward designs have high armholes to give a trim look, but this also gives a slightly restrictive fit. Altering armholes is not a simple task. If the armholes are uncomfortable, the model is not for you.

6. *Sleeves.* Your arms may be different lengths, so always have the tailor measure both arms. Each sleeve (after alterations) should end at the middle of your wristbone. The shirt cuff should extend one half inch beyond the jacket sleeve, which is a good reason to wear a shirt that fits you correctly when you go to buy a suit. (Details on the proper fit of a shirt appear in chapter 8.)

7. *Pattern match.* Here is where manufacturers can cut corners to save money. If you notice a mismatch, so will others. Check the pockets and pocket flaps, the shoulders, the lapel at the point where it is notched, and, most particularly, the long seam down the center of the back.

8. *Vent*. You should look perfect *going* as well as *coming*. To guarantee this, check the vent in the three-way mirror. When you are standing straight, it should lie flat and closed, not gapped or open.

Trousers: Error-Free Fitting

If all points have passed your inspection, the jacket is right. But you are still wearing your old pants. That's the way it should be. There's no use trying on a whole suit if the most important part—the jacket—is wrong. Now you are ready to go to the dressing room and slip on the trousers. As with the jacket, put in your pockets the items that you normally carry.

The popularity of vests waxes and wanes. Currently they are much less in favor than they were in the seventies. The pendulum swings slowly. It will probably be several years before vests are "in" again.

But if the suit has a vest, put it on now. Step up to the three-way mirror, wearing the vest and unaltered trousers. See that the vest covers the waistband of your trousers. No shirt shows, ever, between vest and pants. The fit of a vest should be smooth and close to the body without the least sign of pulling or creasing. If it is patterned, be sure it passes the pattern-match muster.

The bottom button is always left unbuttoned when wearing a vest. I have heard many reasons for this ironbound custom, and am dubious about them all. The story heard most often is that Beau Brummel, the nineteenth-century English dandy, left his bottom button unfastened. The fashionable world figured it must be the proper thing to do and has done it ever since. Whether the story is true or not, I do know it is a gross breach of style to fasten that bottom button.

Better suit manufacturers don't make reversible vests, and the right kind of store doesn't sell them. No matter which way you wear one, it looks wrong.

When trying on trousers, most men are chiefly concerned with the length of each leg. That is the *last* thing for you and the fitter to work on— literally the last, as it should be postponed, ideally, until the second fitting.

Knowing one simple piece of terminology will rate you as an insider.

Most suits have a 6-inch drop. That means that if you wear a size 40 suit, you subtract 6 from 40 and get 34, which is the size of the trousers that go with a 40 suit. Some more highly styled designer and European suits have a 7-inch drop; they are meant for younger, trimmer men. A 7-inch drop on a size 40 suit means that the waist would measure 33. That explains why men who work out and build up their shoulder and neck measurements have difficulty buying suits that fit. Often they wear a size 42 or 43 jacket and have a 33-inch waist—a full 9- or 10-inch drop.

Suits do not come with a 10-inch drop. Men who require it either wear separates (blazers and trousers), have their suits custom-made, or need a truly excellent tailor.

Tailoring of trousers generally involves taking in the center back seam or the two outside seams. If a tailor attempts to create a 10-inch drop from a 6- or 7-inch one, the pants pockets end up way around near the seams. It just doesn't work. Proper tailoring can be done, but it requires almost an entire remake of the trousers. Stores are understandably reluctant to do this. Remember what we said about their having to take back anything that does not suit you? If you were not happy with the work, they would have to "eat" the suit. So if you have a 7- or even 8-inch drop in your measurements, you can get the store to do the proper alterations. But if you require more than that and want to buy your clothes "off the rack," you must have your own tailor do the work.

Unless you are typically proportioned and wear a standard size, your trousers will have to be taken in or let out at the waist and at the rear. For a perfect fit, slip them on without a belt. Position them where you regularly like to wear them. This is important. Don't allow the tailor to adjust them. Sit down; bend over; do the things that will cause stress or slipping. This will allow the trousers to settle naturally and let you judge the fit.

While being fitted, wear the shoes you plan to wear with the new suit. If you have come shopping with shoes that have a slightly different height heel than that of the pair you would wear with the suit, ask the salesman for a pair from the store's stock to wear during the fitting.

Good trousers often come with suspender buttons and almost always have belt loops—loops that are wide enough for a 1¼-inch belt. Keep away from elasticized no-belt styles of pants. They are fine for casual

Steve Varkos (not his real name) is chief fitter at a fine store established seventy years ago in a suburb on Philadelphia's Main Line. His regular customers put themselves in Varkos's hands and it's a smooth fit all around. Steve's virtuoso act is performed when a customer is convinced he knows what's right—and really doesn't know at all. Steve listens and nods, but his chalk has a mind all its own. At the second fitting he is forced to agree when the splendidly suited gentleman gloats, "See, I told you that's how to do it." Some of his accumulated wisdom:

"Nearly two out of three customers need the collar raised, the sleeves made shorter or longer, and that's all. Raising the collar is no problem. Manufacturers of the suits we stock leave enough goods for us to work with. Occasionally we have to lower the collar. Whatever needs doing, we can do.

"Customers have to be brave and face facts. If a man has a big belly, no shoulders and no behind, he's ready for a *portly* model. He'll live through it. That's not the end of the world.

"If one shoulder is higher and the other is lower, a tiny bit of pad comes out of one; a tiny bit goes in the other, and we fix him up. Without surgery. What we never do is cut open the jacket shoulder. You can't close it up again perfectly, no matter how good a tailor you are.

"The different makers have certain ways of cutting clothes. We know this. If I see a customer pulling his pants up or he wants them higher, I tell the salesman to try a Schoeneman on him. The rise of a Schoeneman—the length from the crotch to the top of the waistband—is higher. Some American suits, even the good ones, and most European ones have a short rise.

"Today the best two-button models have a center vent in the back. Some double-breasteds, especially English blazers, have double vents. But my kind of customer, the man who's really on top, wears a single, center vent. So that's what we carry. And some younger men want *no-vent* models. We stock those, too."

weekend or vacation dressing, but they aren't part of the business scene. (Some very fine suits—Paul Stuart's top-of-the-line Canadian models are an example—come without belt loops. When selecting Stuart clothes with an individual client who does not wear suspenders, I always tell the tailor to add belt loops.)

On your return trip to the store to try on the suit after the major alterations have been made, try on the trousers once again. (This time, you have come to the store in the correct shoes.) Repeat your calisthenic-like movements. If there's plenty of room but no slippage, you are ready to address questions of the cuff or no cuff and break or no break.

When you are standing in front of the mirror ready to have the trousers marked for shortening, the tailor will generally say, "Plain bottoms?" as more of a statement than a question. He says this very quickly, because plain bottoms are easier for him to do than cuffs. But if you have been observing how the best-dressed men wear their trousers, you will have him make cuffs.

I know what you are thinking: "Cuffs are for old men; my father wore cuffs." The truth is that well-dressed Ivy League types have always worn cuffs. And now cuffs are back "in" even for the fashion-conscious. If you look at the men's magazines, you will see cuffs. Soon you will be seeing them on more and more men. And your eye will adjust and they will no longer look strange.

You can be sure that the salesman is not going to tell you to choose cuffs. He hopes that you will have the bottoms done in the old way, and then next year, when you see everyone else with cuffs, you will come back for another suit. Remember, if you really hate cuffs, you can always have them taken off. But it's tough to add them. Not impossible, if you save the fabric, but difficult. The current size for cuffs is between 1¼ and 1½ inches.

Managers of better clothing stores in all parts of the country tell me that eight out of ten top executives now wear cuffs. The 20 percent who do not are either freethinkers, mavericks, or not quite up to date. I have been recommending cuffs to my audiences, to the sounds of groans, for several years. Go with cuffs.

Have the fitter measure each leg separately when the pants are in normal position on your waist and you have filled the pockets with the items you normally carry. Legs can vary in length; President Kennedy is said to have worn a half-inch lift on his left heel. Whether you decide on cuffs or

The delicate yet vital matter of *break* or *no break* in the trouser line has been with us since pre–World War II days. Here, reflecting on this dilemma, are fashionable (fictional) young Bertie Wooster and his incomparable butler, Jeeves, as recorded by P. G. Wodehouse in *The Code of the Woosters,* (Doubleday, Doran and Co., 1938).

JEEVES: The trousers perhaps a quarter of an inch higher, sir. One aims at the carelessly graceful break over the instep. It is a matter of the nicest adjustment.

BERTIE WOOSTER: Like that?

JEEVES: Admirable, sir.

WOOSTER: *(Sighing)* There are moments, Jeeves, when one asks oneself, "Do trousers matter?"

JEEVES: The mood will pass, sir.

not, I recommend a slight break in the crease line. The trouser front should rest one quarter to three eighths of an inch on the top of your shoe. And, seen from the side, the bottom should give the illusion of extending downward toward the back. The back of the trouser should approach the top of your shoe heel. It should appear to be about half an inch lower than the front.

John F. Kennedy altered permanently the look of the classic Ivy League suit. Prior to his leading the country in politics—and fashion—the traditional Ivy League jacket had three buttons and a boxy, square cut.

Because JFK's spinal surgery left him wearing a hip brace, he required a suit that would make him appear longer and bigger in the chest, rather than accent the added heaviness of his torso. He had his tailors cut a slightly new style: two buttons instead of the Brooks three . . . a longer line . . . a little bit more accent on the shoulders . . . and a slight suppression in the waist.

Over the ensuing quarter century, the JFK model has become the standard updated style, all but supplanting the three-button tradition.

Accepting or Rejecting the Suit:
Checking the Final Fit

On the day you are scheduled to pick up the suit or come in for the second (with luck, final) fitting, wear a shirt and collar that complement the suit, and wear the right shoes.

If you are not completely sure of your sense of fit, try to bring someone with you who is. You will be as critical as possible in assessing the tailor's work, but after all, it's you you'll be looking at. Another pair of eyes—objective ones—often spot a wrinkle or a bulge in the back that your own inspection might let slip by. If you cannot bring the right person with you, try on the suit for him or her soon afterward; then return it to the store for any further changes.

Check to see that all the alterations were made. And were they made flawlessly? Was the collar raised? Were the trousers taken in? Those are the questions you are there to have answered. The mirror will tell you. Transfer everything from the pockets of your old suit to the new one and see if the lines are still smooth. Bend; stretch; sit down.

Closely examine the lapels and chest. No trace of interfacing—no ridges—should be visible beneath the fabric. (Again, interfacing is the canvaslike stiffener between layers of fabric.) That's very important, because any slight unevenness will be magnified as weeks go by, and will seriously mar the jacket's appearance after a dozen or so wearings. This is one reason you may not always see what you are paying for when you buy a good suit. The quality of a good suit, with much hand stitching, lies within, and becomes evident over time.

Seven-year-old Marco Salvi (not his real name) sat on the floor of a tailor shop, sewing the same stitch over and over on a piece of scrap fabric. He was learning the process called *overcasting,* used on the seam inside a pants leg.

This was Italy just after World War II, and good fabric was scarce. After Marco completed a row of stitches, he would show them to his father, the master tailor, get a nod of approval, then rip them out and start over.

Today, his name shortened to Marc, he is master fitter and head tailor at a fine men's store in Hennepin County, Minnesota.

Income levels run uncommonly high in Hennepin. It is a residential area favored by Minneapolis financial and communications executives.

Between fittings one afternoon, his tape measure draped around his neck, Marc Salvi took time to express these random thoughts.

· I always ask the customer, "How do you like the sleeves? About here?" Some say they want them shorter. Some say longer. I say, "Good. Maybe just a quarter inch longer; what do you think?" Whatever they tell me, I do. But if they leave it up to me, I'll do it exactly right. My regular customers do that—they leave it to me.

· I see younger men come in who have tremendous shoulders from their workouts and their tennis. Big shoulders and chest. The rest of them, mostly their behind, is too small for their coat size. I've got a tough problem. But one way or the other, they will wind up with a perfect fit.

· When you buy some lower-quality suits, there's a tape inside the lapels on the edges, and also on the outer edges of the coat. The tape shrinks after a year; maybe even sooner. The suit wrinkles. On a good suit, that doesn't happen.

· On the best suits, the top of the line, the manufacturer sends us matching thread. When we do alterations, it's a perfect match.

· When I see a customer try on a gabardine, I look quick to see if it's basically a good fit. If it isn't, we try to show him something else. Gabardine weave is tight, very tight. Any seams we open might show. It's not meant for big alterations, like on a tweed or soft woolen.

· The toughest customer? The short guy. He doesn't trust the tailor. He's afraid I'll make him look . . . short. Tall guys never give you a hard time. They look in the mirror; they like what they see.

Be wary of the fitter's and salesman's assurances that "we'll take care of that right away" when you point out a crease or an imbalance in the sides of the jacket. That's precisely what you don't want them to do—take care of it by *pressing* it. Shape is not built into suits by steaming and forcing the fabric. Sewing is required, and sewing is what you should insist on. Most likely, everything will have gone well, and only the cuffs—if they have not been done—must be added before the suit can be picked up. But if you are dissatisfied, insist that the flaw be reworked, not merely pressed. If you don't find perfection, you haven't found the right store, and nothing less will do.

The When and Why of
Returning a Suit

Let's suppose that things went wrong during the fitting and trying-on processes. The jacket seems pinched. It pulls together too tightly when buttoned, and there are horizontal stress lines across the middle. They are slight, and they disappear if you suck in your breath, but they exist.

The fitter, tailor, and head salesman gather around. They eye the coat carefully, pass their hands over it frequently, admire the unexcelled workmanship and success of the alterations. They assure you it is perfect. "Would we let you walk out of here if it wasn't perfect?" they ask.

They've put their collective finger right on it. Would they, indeed? It depends on the store, your relationship to it, and the reality concerning the "flaw." My experience tells me that in an absolutely first-class establishment, one in which you are recognized as a good customer, the scope or the importance of the objection doesn't signify. They want you to be completely satisfied, and if the problem can't be worked out, they will "eat" the suit and start over.

You needn't worry about the store's indigestion. They have enough clout with the manufacturer to pass the problem back to him. He'll take back the goods, issue a credit to the store, and shrug it off.

The real worry occurs when the script takes a different turn—when the store's personnel persuade you, against your strong belief, that the jacket is perfect and that you'll gain compliments whenever you appear in the suit. You take it home, yet the first time you wear it you are unhappy, and the second and third times confirm your dissatisfaction. The suit just doesn't fit right.

My firm advice: Take it back. You have worn it three times too many. Don't talk to the salesman or anyone except the manager. Tell him firmly that you objected all along, were talked into accepting it (which, you admit, you never should have done), and cannot—will not—ever wear this suit again. Period.

In a department store you'll have little or no real trouble. You will receive a credit on your charge account. You are free to buy your suit elsewhere, although you may have reason to stick with them and be doubly vigilant this time. A specialty store may issue a refund if you are firm and unyielding. More often, however, the best you can do there is receive a complete credit and a chance to start over. Tip: Do not pick the same model, or even the same maker. That cut hasn't worked well for you once, and it probably won't a second time, either. Keep away from it.

If you bought the suit during an "absolutely no returns" sale, there may be little you can do, though some of the better stores will accommodate you even then. You are equally out of luck if you bought it in a discount house.

Experience is the name everyone gives to his mistakes.

—OSCAR WILDE

Of course, I don't make the same mistakes twice. The second time, I make *different* mistakes.

—LAURA LAUER

One thing you should never do is wear a suit that bothers you. If you feel it doesn't fit or detracts from your image, don't wear it. If discarding it entails a financial loss, of course that hurts. But the loss of confidence, and subsequently of power, hurts infinitely more. Using the principles in this chapter, you are not likely to incur a dollar loss. But if there is one, call it part of the price of learning.

7

Life at the Top:
The Custom-Made Suit

Custom-Made: There's Nothing Like It

There is a whole world of suits and suit making in which the atmosphere is considerably rarefied, even more so than that of the first-class stores we've been talking about. It is the timeless world of bespoke tailoring, where you are measured—every inch of you—consulted by the tailor about such details as the width of lapels and dimensions of pocket flaps, and get to try on a hand-sewn masterpiece every step of the way.

Current prices of custom-made suits in fine old establishments: J. Press in New Haven will make you a two-piece model cut along their Ivy League, natural shoulder lines—or any variation of it that you specify—for $1,250 and up. Their brochure de-

76

scribes their service as "starting from scratch with a choice of superfine British Woolens and Worsteds; next, a personal cutting pattern reflects individual measurements, stature characteristics and style preference; the clothes then receive the hand craftmanship of a journeyman tailor and expert fittings by a master tailor until complete." These suits require several fittings.

Bespoke suits in your choice of a perfectly splendid fabric—the finest of imported luxury suitings—at one of the true custom tailors still in business across the nation, run slightly more than the Press suit in New Haven. You'll get the very best, but don't be surprised if your bill approaches $1,400.

Do I recommend custom-made suits? No, unless you have a severe fit problem. Otherwise, maybe eight or ten years from now, when dressing for excellence is an established way of life for you, and when more than a thousand dollars for a suit (if prices have stayed at that level) is within your range.

Made-to-Measure: A Cut Above the Rest

Nowadays the tailor who will make a suit from scratch is a rarity. Easier to find, and a more realistic choice when fitting is a problem or when a splurge is indicated, is a *made-to-measure* suit. (This is often called special order.)

Made-to-measure is a category that falls between the luxury of bespoke tailoring and the utility of off-the-rack, ready-made clothing. Only the better manufacturers—Hickey-Freeman, Oxxford, and their peers—can do the job right. In fact, the majority of suit makers will not attempt it. And only a superior store—one with a topflight fitter on staff—can transmit the right specifications to the factory. Fortunately, the number of those stores seems to be increasing.

At Barneys and Tripler's in New York City and at Neiman-Marcus and Saks Fifth Avenue in all their branches across the country, special-order suits are all in the same price range, depending on fabric. You'll pay $700 to $900 for a Porsche or Maserati among suits.

Made-to-measure suits are expensive, but nowhere near the stratospheric prices of custom-made clothing. You can figure that you will pay about $200 more than the regular price of a suit to have it cut to your requirements.

Paul Ostrove, vice-president of Paul Stuart's clothing store, told me that even if a man is not a difficult fit, there are other good reasons to go the made-to-measure route. A customer may have a specific pattern, color, or fabric that he particularly wants in order to round out his wardrobe. If he has in mind a dark gray glen plaid with a faint burgundy line, he may come up against a blank wall in every store where he looks. But the swatch books will have it.

Ostrove, whose store does a heavy volume in made-to-measures, went on to describe a customer who might even be an easy fit, but whose favorite old suit has seen better days. It is time to replace it; however, this season his regular store does not have that same pattern. Another possibility is that he has decided he would like the trousers made with pleats. He'll get what he wants on a special order.

Making a special order, or made-to-measure, suit jacket is not as involved as having one custom-made. If a 41 long is basically your size, for instance, the fitter will work with that. He will carefully indicate if one shoulder must be raised and shortened; the collar raised; the sleeve lengths changed; and the back expanded on the left and taken in on the right. At the factory, when the order is received, they don't alter an existing jacket. Instead, they make adjustments for a size 41 long and cut the suit to your specifications. If you need a size 32 trouser (a 9-inch drop from the jacket, and impossible to find ready-made), they make it. In eight weeks or so, the suit arrives at your store. You try on the semifinished jacket and trousers. Any further adjustments are noted, and a final try-on, a week or so later, should reveal a perfection you had never thought you'd see in a three-way mirror.

Occasionally that perfection is delayed. The manufacturer appears to have ignored some of the measurements or may have adjusted them faultily, and the results are not what they should be. When you try on the suit at your first fitting, everyone knows this. The store salesman who is getting credit for the sale may say the suit looks terrific; so may the store's tailor. But they know it does not fit. You can be sure of that.

Inwardly they expect you to insist that it be done correctly. If you care enough to give them this special order, the suit should not merely look good, it should be perfect. Insist on it.

That Hong Kong Tailor

A question that is almost always asked at every Wardrobe Engineering seminar is, "What about those ads I see for custom-made suits from Hong Kong? They're supposed to be great. And the ads say the whole job will cost only $300."

My answer usually is, "Wait until the next time you're in Hong Kong. And then, I'd caution you to be careful."

You know the kind of ad they're referring to: one that announces the arrival of a world-famous master tailor, now on a United States tour, direct from Hong Kong. He'll be in suite 235 of the Ramada Inn in your town on Tuesday and Wednesday of next week.

From what I've seen, the fabrics are inferior to those in a good American suit, the tailoring is spotty, and the fit is a toss-up—you might win or you might lose. My advice: Don't knock on the door of suite 235.

A footnote that illustrates the point: I met an attractive, well-dressed Oriental man and woman who were visiting the States. I'd been told they were extremely wealthy. He said he always buys suits off the rack when he is here, but only from our top-of-the-line manufacturers. He told me that America's top ready-mades have tailoring far superior to suits custom-made in the Orient. And he lives there.

London's Incomparable Tailoring

If you are ready now for a touch of incomparable elegance, consider having a suit made in a Savile Row shop in London's West End. Of course, you've got to get to England first, but the money you save by buying there instead of at home might pay your plane fare. And the quiet atmosphere, dark wood cabinets, and bolts of soft woolens in themselves have aesthetic value. So paying $500–$600 for a $1,000 suit is quite inviting. And your cost per wearing will be minuscule, since the suit will probably outlast all your others. The fit will be extraordinary, unlike any you have experienced. I'm sure you'll be answering inquiries with, "Oh, this? I picked it up in London, and have been wearing it steadily for at least a dozen years."

One drawback: waiting for the fittings. Although there are two shops on Savile Row (Anderson & Sheppard and Gieves & Hawkes) that can turn out extraordinary products within a week of taking your measurements, most bespoke tailors require a month or so. Among the very best: Kilgour, French & Stanley; Huntsman; Hawes & Curtis.

PART II

—

PUTTING TOGETHER THE LOOK THAT WINS

8

The Finishing Touch:
The Art of Coordinating
Shirts and Ties

Howard T. is assistant director of data processing for the entire southern region of his huge company. He couldn't wait to collar me during the preseminar coffee session at a conference room in Nashville. "A couple of weeks ago I bought six shirts. The week before that, I spent two hours on Saturday buying half a dozen ties. And nothing goes with anything!"

There wasn't time right then to tell Howard what he *should have done*. Instead, along with his Danish, he got sympathy and reassurance that he's far from the first man to suffer that particular frustration—and a promise that within the next two hours he would have an absolute antidote.

Here, straight off, is the solution to Howard's problem: *Buy shirts and ties as combination units, not separately.* How can you possibly keep in mind the colors and patterns of six shirts while inspecting a store full of ties of every possible color, texture, and design? You can't. Nobody can.

Buy one shirt. When you do, wear the suit that you have in mind for it. If that's not convenient, bring along a piece of the suiting fabric that was left over when your trousers were altered. Suppose the shirt is a cotton tab collar with muted burgundy stripes on a white background. It works perfectly with your medium dark gray suit, the one cut along traditional American lines (single-breasted and soft-shouldered). Now buy precisely the tie that will add flair, color, and *authority* to the combination. It might be a silk charcoal gray and burgundy foulard.

Whatever your first tie selection, immediately choose a second one. It might be a much less conservative design than the gray silk one, perhaps a paisley or a bold stripe. Fine—now you can satisfy either of two contradictory moods.

With those two ties in hand, go back to the shirt counter. If you see another shirt—say, a blue cotton broadcloth—that's right for the suit, buy it. Either one of your two ties *might* work well with it. But *might* isn't

---

Compounding Your Clothing Investment

When you buy a suit, shirt, and tie combination, the overwhelmingly heavy portion of your outlay goes for the suit. If the total is $565, with the suit costing $500, a $40 shirt accounts for 7 percent and a $25 tie is only 4 percent of your total cost.

By buying a few extra shirts and ties, your possibilities for exciting, nonboring appearances are increased geometrically. Just think: With 1 suit, 8 shirts, and 15 ties, you will have 120 different combinations. Impressed?

Among the shirts you might consider: a dressy white; a white button-down; a light blue pinpoint; a dressy solid blue; oxford cloth and end-on-end blue button-downs; and two to four various stripes.

good enough. You're out to choose clothes that call out "perfection." You want to be one of those guys who are recognized as flawless—an important person every day of the week. So select another tie or two right at that moment, specifically for your new blue broadcloth shirt.

I don't urge you to go on a binge and buy four or five shirts and ten ties to go with them. Those kinds of expenditures and decisions can be overwhelming if you are hit with them all in one afternoon. But buying two or three shirts and a couple of ties for each is a sensible goal for one day's trip to the stores.

A Very Comfortable Thing

"A clean shirt," thought Oliver, *"is a very comfortable thing, very."* Comfort may have been at the front of Oliver Twist's mind, and I don't downplay its importance. But your relationship to a shirt—the right shirt—is even more critical for your overall image. For a full day, an important day in the business world you inhabit, it is going to frame your face. It is up front, the focus of your associates' attention. Your face is exclusively *you.* And your face is set off by, framed by, and an adjunct of, your shirt.

Not long ago an "authority" on dressing for business success published another book on dress. In it, he advocates wearing colored shirts and tweed suits for normal business wear. Save your navy suit and white shirts for special dress-up occasions, he says. I couldn't disagree more strenuously.

Which part of your life influences most heavily where and who you will be ten years from now? Who has the most impact on your life: the pleasant fellows you'll chat with at Sunday's cocktail party or the associates and superiors you see at the office?

In my book, saving your Sunday best for Sundays is unwise. Come as close to perfection as you can from Monday straight through to Friday. If you have a breakfast meeting planned, you can dress impressively for it and be dressed correctly for anything that occurs during that day. Wear the right shirt and tie to the office and you can accept that last-minute invitation to a concert, knowing you're dressed appropriately for after eight, too.

A navy suit and white shirt are not too dressy for most business circumstances. But given a navy suit, it is just one way to go. Your choices are infinitely wider than that perennial classic; these pages will describe dozens of choices and combinations. I do want to stress, though, that the "banker's special" is not only for bankers; it most certainly is appropriate for managers in marketing, manufacturing, retailing, insurance, and just about any facet of industry. Its popularity in investment and financial circles is logical. When you are dealing with people's money, they want to think of you as stable, dependable, and confident. A navy blue suit and white shirt say all that.

One Blue Suit—Three Different People

The versatility of a good dark blue suit is brought home strikingly when you consider how you would appear wearing the same suit with:
- a white broadcloth shirt with a standard point collar, and a navy tie with a small, gray pattern
- a pale blue pinpoint oxford shirt with a tab collar, and a regimental striped tie in red and blue
- a yellow oxford shirt with a button-down collar, and a paisley tie with yellow, light blue, and navy predominating.

Would a field engineer wear the "presidential combination," all crisp contrast in navy and white, on a plant visit? Emphatically not. A flannel suit, a blazer, or a tweed sports jacket would make more sense. There might be times when khaki or corduroy pants would be logical choices. But when he is meeting with the plant manager and intends to introduce some innovative ideas, the blue suit and white shirt look may be a tool that adds weight to his suggestions.

Collars—Right and Wrong

The collar is where most men run into problems when buying a shirt, although not because their faces are too long or their chins are too sharp to accommodate a certain style of collar. Any reasonable variation of the five basic collars—*regular* (also called straight or point), *pin* (including a variation called the eyelet because of the small holes through which the collar pin extends), *tab, button-down,* and *spread*—can be worn by anyone.

When problems occur, it is because (1) the collar is too tight or too roomy, or (2) it reflects the wrong degree of formality for the suit or occasion, or (3) it has too slick or too fashion-forward a look for your industry or your personality.

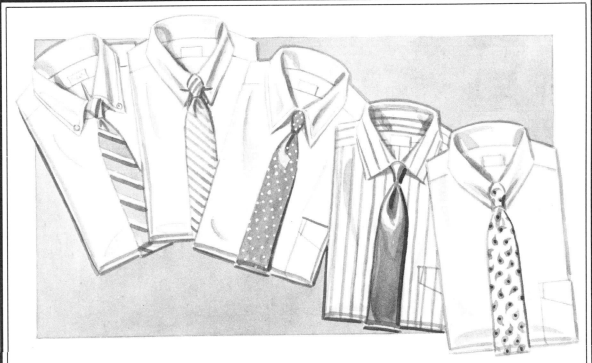

Shirt collar styles *(left to right):* button-down; point collar worn with a collar pin; point collar; spread collar; tab collar

If Clint Eastwood wears his collar unbuttoned, with or without a tie covering the gap, that's because he's a superstar and his role calls for it. If you unbutton your collar for comfort at your desk, it's probably because you are wearing the wrong size collar. If you are like a huge percentage of businessmen, you consistently order shirt collars that are one half to one inch too small. You doom yourself to too-tight, uncomfortable shirts. They're literally a pain in the neck.

And they look terrible, even when buttoned, because they squeeze an overlapping of flesh up around the top of the collar.

Why does this happen? Because time passes. Six years ago Bert wore a 15½ neck size. Six long years went by, and Bert's neck gained a half inch, but Bert says, "I've worn a 15½/34 shirt all my life." He still buys 15½ collars. In the car on the way home he's got to open that button, and most days in the office he does it by three o'clock. He thinks it is the laundry's fault. Or, now that he has progressed to wearing all-cotton shirts, he blames the tight collars on shrinkage.

Bert, get with it! Move up to a size 16 collar.

The charts on pages 136–139 outline the "formality ratios" among various styles of shirts and suits. A classic straight collar is perfectly right with all suits and sports jackets. Equally correct, and only a shade more formal, are a pin collar and a tab collar. Although many people seem not to realize it, a button-down collar is *less* formal than the others. It is not quite dressy enough for a pinstripe or double-breasted suit. There are, however, extremely well-dressed men who exhibit what I call the Eastern Seaboard Syndrome. They are perfectly comfortable in button-down shirts at all times—even with the dressiest pinstripe suits. Don't follow their lead, however, if you want to be on target in your clothing choices.

Spread collars are a variation of the straight point, but they are much more suited to evening/social wear than to business. Many of the executives I dress move in the highest corporate circles. If that's where you're bound, I don't recommend spread collars; they sometimes convey a message of glamour that you want to avoid. But if you are convinced that you are at your best in a spread collar, then that's the one for you.

The newer, smaller fashion-forward collars, seen on some shirts by Giorgio Armani, Calvin Klein, and Ralph Lauren, are fine for weekend and social wear, but should be approached with caution for office wear. Again, be alert against a dandyish, glamorous image that is inappropriate for most industries.

Choice Factors Among Shirts

Color, pattern, and collar style constitute the big decision factors when you are shopping for shirts. They are discretionary and, once determined, pretty well narrow down the selection. The remaining factors to consider, before the essential matter of *fit,* are:

· **Fabrics.** Your choice for business dress is uncomplicated: choose all cotton or cotton and polyester. Pure cotton is classic, luxurious, expensive, and requires ironing. However, if you can afford the slightly higher initial cost and the upkeep, that's the way to go. I am convinced that men who are headed for the top pay the extra cost for all-cotton shirts, and find the time to locate the best laundry around. Their shirts are

---

A Blue Chip Investment

Occasionally when I consult with men in large companies, I hear a pattern emerge. More than one man says to me, "What I'd really like is if you could make me look like . . ." and they name one of their colleagues. The most recent of these was a man in the company whom I had not met. When I asked someone what it was about this man that had prompted three managers to want to look like him, the answer was a surprising and interesting one: "He pays meticulous attention to how his shirts are ironed."

It was hard to believe. All were high-powered executives earning well into the six figures, yet what they envied about one of their colleagues was the crispness of his shirts! I finally met this man and found it was true. His shirt *was* perfect, and to add to the neat appearance, he wore a collar pin. When I mentioned how much he was admired by his colleagues, he told me he knew that he was not a tall, prepossessing figure; in fact, he admitted to being a bit on the portly side. But he knew it was important to have a crisp look, so he had his shirts done by the best laundry in town.

Moral: Having your shirts laundered is a business investment very much worth pursuing.

ironed properly. Collars and cuffs are crisp and creaseless, with no wrinkles across the chest, and the starched-stiff look is blessedly absent. I sometimes see young men who are aware of the new popularity of all-cotton fabrics, but who feel they can do the ironing themselves and no one will know. Everyone knows. Laundering is a job for a professional.

If wash-and-wear is the only practical route for you—and remember, they, too, require some slight ironing for a perfect look—confine your selections to blends with a lower, rather than higher, percentage of synthetic yarn. High polyester content retains perspiration odors. The synthetic yarn will eventually form little "pills" on the shirt's surface which are distracting and unpleasant.

· **Weaves.** *Broadcloth* has a tight construction that makes it smooth, soft, rich, and somewhat formal. When woven of long-staple Sea Island cotton, it is the most luxurious of domestic fabrics. *Pinpoint oxford cloth* is a tightly woven fabric, somewhat similar to classic oxford but much finer and dressier. You almost need a magnifying glass to see the oxford

---

One Expert's Opinion

The weave of the familiar button-down oxford cloth shirt makes it look too lifeless. *The texture affects the color.* It, in turn, gives the individual who's wearing it a drab, if not dull, look. Although it is one of the most widely accepted shirts for a businessman to wear, it deprives him of a finished, attractive, and professional look.

We have been conditioned to think that the blue oxford cloth shirt gives a youthful look. But actually it makes men look older and generally more tired.

By substituting the newer shirt fabric, blue *pinpoint* oxford cloth, the whole effect is changed, giving a more vital and attractive look. You get the benefit of the traditional oxford look but in a much more complimentary and youthful way.

—SANDRA MERRILL HERSCOTT,
Authority on color,
Boston Architectural Center

weave. It is made of the finest cotton yarns, which brings the price up ten to fifteen dollars over the cost of a regular oxford cloth shirt. It is worth the difference.

Oxford cloth, that ever-present necessity for Ivy League button-down shirts, is a looser, more open weave. Equally adaptable to all cotton or cotton and polyester blends, it has a slightly casual look and feel. As a shirting fabric, a wide range of colors is acceptable: white, blue, yellow, pink, ivory, gray, and even lilac. *End-on-end* is the phrase used to describe the material of fine pastel shirts—light blues, pinks, and creams. Colored threads are interwoven with white ones, in a fabric similar to oxford cloth. *Chambray, satin stripes, jacquard* and *white-on-white* (a variation of jacquard) are specialty weaves, described on page 139, and not appropriate for most business wear.

· **Cuts.** There are three cuts, or tapers, available in ready-made shirts. (Most manufacturers confine their products to one style; if you find a new shirt by Gant, Hathaway, Troy Guild, or R. & O. Hawick congenial, try to find others by the same maker. They all will be cut on the same pattern.) A *full-cut* shirt that is loose and commodious enough for the large-boned or portly man or for one who simply prefers a conservative, Brooks Brothers look. *Regular-cut,* or semifitted, is slightly trimmer; less full throughout the body. *Fitted* shirts, also called body shirts, are severely tapered at the waist. European "designer" shirts cut along Italian lines are almost always tapered markedly, with the shoulder much wider than the waist. The newer emphasis on large cuts is influencing American designers to cut their shirts much more fully than previously: Perry Ellis, Andrew Fezza, and Ralph Lauren are setting the style.

· **Cuffs.** Conventional single-button cuffs are known as *barrel cuffs.* Today, some shirt makers add a second button, lined up horizontally about three fourths of an inch farther along the cuff. More about that later. Cuffs with two buttonholes and no buttons, which require cuff links, are known as *French cuffs.* They are a touch more formal and dressy. Both are acceptable, and the choice is purely a matter of personal preference.

· **Collar pins and tabs.** Tab collars require a collar button to give them their distinctive, ultraneat shape. Shirts designed to be worn with a pin have a small eyelet sewn into each collar point. Buy a simple bar of

Reading Shirt Cuts

Alert observers can "read" the cut of a businessman's shirt. Here are some widely held perceptions:

- Full-cut shirts are worn by men who are set in their ways. They have been raised in elite circles and know that "a gentleman wears a full-cut shirt." They also may be older men who have earned a bit of a paunch along the way, and choose a loose, full effect to minimize it.
- Regular-cut shirts are indicators of a traditional, middle-of-the-road personality. He's the new establishment. Although he's receptive to new ideas and not stodgy, he's not ready for anything he considers extreme. You always know where you stand with a guy like this.
- Flair, daring, and a touch of exhibitionism: Those are the characteristics of the man in the fitted shirt that hugs his slim, flat-stomached body like a second skin. The shirt is rarely a white one. His choice runs to patterns, bold stripes, and designer labels. He seeks to be perceived as a swinging, with-it fellow, right on the cutting edge of fashion. Successful executives do not dress this way.
- Tacky and makeshift is what knowledgeable observers think about shirts altered with darts (tucks sewn into too-full shirts to make them more tapered at the waist). The best shirts are slightly full in the body—not enormous, but somewhat full. For a smoother fit for any shirt use the "military school tuck": fold the side of the shirt to the back, as you'd do when folding sharp corners on a bed sheet.

unadorned gold or silver with ball or cube tips to insert in the eyelets. If you like the collar pin look, you can use a slide-on bar with any shirt that has a regular point collar.

- **Stays.** If your new shirt requires stays—small, flat strips of plastic or metal slipped inside the collar points to make them lie flat—it is important that they be removable. Permanent stays, stitched inside the collar, invariably cause creases when the shirt is pressed. Or worse, they melt and fuse to the collar. Reject any shirt from which you cannot extract the stays before laundering.

· **Monograms.** Many men like monograms. Others don't. It is totally a matter of preference. But if you do choose to show your initials on your shirt, certain guidelines exist. *Discreet* is the operative word. Showy monograms are in a league with diamond pinky rings.

The lettering should be small—not much over one fourth of an inch in height—and set in a straight line. The letters should be in the order of first, middle, and last name, and embroidered in medium blue, navy, or black.

Monograms are worn in one of two places. First choice is a few inches above the belt on the left side. This may sound strange, but it is correct, and a strong first choice. Second choice is on the upper part of the pocket. There is no third choice; a monogrammed cuff is too showy a placement, and a monogrammed collar is unspeakably gauche.

A monogram implies that a shirt is custom-made. Indeed, the elegant shirts worn by Robert A. Meister, vice-chairman of Fred S. James & Co., are made for him by one of the finest shops in Europe. One of his most handsome shirts is cut of pale blue cloth woven in a subtle mini-herringbone pattern. Bob prefers French cuffs. His monogram is placed unobtrusively above his belt line, embroidered in blue a shade deeper than the shirt.

· **Short sleeves.** In business dress they don't exist. Successful executives do not wear short sleeves under suit jackets. Nor do they regard as a serious person anyone seen wearing short-sleeved dress shirts. "But what about the summer months?" some men ask me. Still the same: long sleeves only. But I tell them they will be much more comfortable in long-sleeved 100 percent cotton shirts, which breathe and release body heat. (Sure, they need ironing. That's why laundries were invented—and you *can* afford to send out your best shirts.)

Measurements the Accurate Way

Sports shirts are manufactured with "average" sleeve lengths: small, medium, and large. Dress shirts fit for office wear are marked with specific neck and sleeve sizes: a 15-inch neck and 33-inch sleeve, for example.

Traditionally, shirt makers produced a full range of sizes in every style and color. The better manufacturers still do, running from 14½/32, 14½/33, 15/32, 15/33, 15/34, and 15/35 on up through 17½/36. Collar measurements are in half-inch progressions; sleeve lengths are in full inches. But some manufacturers have hit on a way to cut corners. They call it the "adjustable" sleeve length. It eliminates their need to produce shirts in every size. They make just two sleeve lengths—designated 32–33 and 34–35. So instead of four accurately fitting 15s, you are given a choice of two, neither of which is likely to be precisely your size. Here is where the "adjustable" feature comes in. An additional button has been sewn on the cuff allowing the wearer to tighten or loosen the cuff. This partially compensates for the sloppiness of the fit. It also announces to the world that you are wearing a second-rate shirt.

Find a store that sells shirts made by fine manufacturers, offering a full range of sizes. Be aware that even the best makers' sizes tend to vary, one from another. A size 15 collar in a Hathaway shirt might be looser or tighter than a size 15 Gant or John Henry.

Manufacturers' differences notwithstanding, there is only one way to measure a collar. Using a tape measure, holding it around your neck where the top of the collar should be. Better yet, go into a fine store and ask the salesperson to measure you.

Beating the "Adjustable" Shirt Dodge

My advice is to stay away from the double-button cuff, alias the adjustable shirt. Buy fine shirts that come in actual sizes.

But if you are a 32½ or 34½ sleeve size—the actual length of those 32–33 and 34–35 combos—and happen across an adjustable shirt that you really like, here's what to do. Wear the shirt and determine which is the correct button. Cut off the other one. Save it in case you lose a button. Now the world will never know that you did not buy the very best.

Sleeves are measured with the arm extending down and bent slightly at the elbow. The sleeve length is measured in inches beginning from the center of the back, just under the collar, over the shoulder, and down past the elbow to the bottom of the wristbone. Normally, sleeves run from 32 to 36 inches.

Once you find a reliable manufacturer whose shirts fit you well, one large enough to offer a wide choice of fabrics and styles, try to stick with his label. Sleeves will be long enough to show the requisite half inch of "linen" beyond your jacket sleeve. Collars won't squeeze or flap around your neck.

How to Recognize Quality Construction

Most men separate first-rate shirts from merely good ones by noting several obvious distinctions. Number one—too often, the only one—is the name of the manufacturer. The label tells it all, they say. I'm not so sure. It tells a lot. But nothing is forever, and standards change. The second and third widely noticed criteria are, "Is the shirt all cotton?" and "Does the cloth feel rich?" If all three factors pass muster, they figure the shirt is worth the premium price it bears. And it might very likely be.

Here, however, are six hallmarks of quality in shirts that clothing experts look for. They are specific, easily discerned, and nearly always an infallible guide to excellence in shirting.

- The shirt is long—it extends at least nine inches below the trouser top. Because it is full length, it has seven buttons. Manufacturers who cut corners need only six on their skimpy, short-tailed products.
- The yoke—a panel at the top of the back that runs from shoulder to shoulder—is split. That is, it has a vertical seam running up its center, which makes for a much better fit. No one's back is straight as a board; his shirt shouldn't be flat, either. A split yoke might at first glance appear to be a cost-cutting trick for using smaller pieces of fabric. Actually it requires more tailoring and adds to the manufacturing cost.
- If patterned, the woven design elements mesh perfectly at the front seams and at the pocket.

- The sleeve opening has a button halfway up its length. The buttonhole is cut through a placket, or seamed band, a miniature version of the band which runs down the front of the shirt.
- Buttons are made of mother-of-pearl or bone, never plastic. They are sewn with a secure cross-stitch, not merely two parallel rows of machine stitching.
- Single-needle tailoring, if claimed by the manufacturer, is your assurance that the seams will not pull apart or unravel.

An Intriguing Custom

A considerable number of my days are spent in an absolutely ideal way. I accompany a wealthy, clothes-conscious man—often a top executive of a leading corporation—as we shop the finest stores and spend *his* money. On *him*. He defers to my judgment, accepts nearly all my suggestions, and is grateful that things work out as well as they do. His company pays a significant fee for the day's consultation. These are busy men; their time is valuable and must be used judiciously. Because I spend considerable time preselecting items that will suit their needs, we can cover much ground in a short time.

Nearly half these men tell me they have to wear custom-made shirts. Over the years, I have come to recognize a man who is so knowledgeable about clothes that he requires the subtleties and sophistication of a true custom shirt. Yet some men, particularly in the higher echelons of investment and accounting firms, definitely do not want any noticeable touches apart from the expected. They consider many custom flourishes to be affectations. But they have been influenced by some salesman or writer on the need to wear so-called custom-made shirts. When I ask them why, their answer is usually that they wear an off-size sleeve length—32¼ or 34½. This does not necessitate buying a custom-made shirt. (In a moment I will explain exactly what is a better course in those cases.)

Some stores claim that a custom shirt, made in "our own shop," is only a few dollars more than a ready-made shirt. And during sale periods, the custom-made may actually cost less. Now, I ask you, does this make sense? If you were in the shirt business, could it possibly cost no more to make one shirt to specific measurements than to make one of thousands in a factory? Of course not. Something has to give.

Generally that something is the fabric. Another something is even more basic. In most instances they are not offering you a true *custom-made* shirt. It is a *made-to-measure,* or semicustom, shirt, one on which adjustments are made to a stock pattern.

In the real thing twelve or thirteen separate measurements are taken. An individual muslin (thin cotton) pattern is cut and fitted on the customer before the actual fabric is touched. The entire shirt is made by one craftsman to fit one specific customer. The amount of work involved in this procedure would not justify using less than the finest fabrics. And the prices reflect it. True custom-made shirts cost $90 to well over $100, and a minimum order of four at a time is required.

Made-to-measure shirts start at "special" prices of $38.50 and run up to nearly $100, depending on the fabric you choose. And the fabric you like and choose is never the one that costs $38.50.

If You Work in New York, Dallas, or Austin . . .

"The successful businessman is in a hurry," says Richard Contratti, whose made-to-measure shirt service is highly thought of by New York's Wall Street crowd. "He doesn't have time to spend hunting for the special shirts he wants. Also, the consistency factor is important. The difference between an ordinary shirt and a fine one is in the quality of the fabric and the craftsmanship. We use better quality cotton and our craftsmanship is always consistent."

Mr. Contratti provides a unique service. He makes fine shirts to measure for his customers, and he goes to their offices with swatches of fabric. Once a customer is established and his measurements on file, an appointment may take only a few minutes. Several weeks later—usually about four—the completed shirts are delivered. The cost ranges from $45 to $85 without monograms.

Richard Contratti's office is at 79 Luddington Road, West Orange, NJ 07052, (201) 736-7627. He also has offices in Dallas and Austin.

I usually recommend to my clients that we go to the finest store in town and select shirts and ties that are right there on the shelves. No need to be your own designer, to make decisions about which cut, collar, fabric, and color you want. No waiting four to six weeks for a shirt you can use tomorrow. You have the actual shirt in front of you to work with when coordinating it with your suit and tie. There's no need to visualize what the collar style will actually look like. And no surprise problem if the dye lot turns out to be a tone or two off when the final product is delivered.

But what about the half-inch differential in the sleeve size, which is the reason behind my client's claim that he can't buy ready-made shirts? That is easily remedied. If he requires a 33½ sleeve, we buy a size 34. The store's alteration department will shorten the sleeve half an inch. Fine stores offer this service. Some do the work for free; more often there is a $5 charge. The work can be done from the shoulder or the cuff, but it is not advisable to shorten a sleeve more than two inches. The sleeve proportions would be thrown off and the shirt's total appearance would seem out of sync.

However, you might have reasons for ordering a specially made shirt. One reason might be that you cannot find a certain fabric in a ready-made shirt. Another could be that you like French cuffs on shirts made of fabrics that are not highly dressy. Most often, stores carry French cuffs on only their dressiest designs. You might want a hairline or Bengal

C. F. Hathaway, the noted shirt maker, recently conducted a survey of 2,300 CEOs, presidents, and key vice-presidents of leading corporations; 1,200 responded.

These facts emerged:
• 73 percent of the executives buy shirts for themselves, and wives play a role in shirt purchases for 44 percent. (The total exceeds 100 percent because some gave alternate responses.)
• The average number of dress shirts bought in one year's time is eight.
• Given a choice of collars and fabrics in a free shirt, 47 percent chose button-down, 53 percent opted for straight; 45 percent chose all cotton, 54 percent chose a blend.

stripe, or even a pinpoint oxford, with a French cuff. You may also like the tony look of a dress shirt made without a pocket.

Or you might have a short neck. You may need a shirt with a low slope (a collar that measures not much more than an inch at the back). If you know what you want and are prepared to wait for it and pay for it, why not? Keep in mind that the minimum order is nearly always four. Custom-made or made-to-measure may be the way to go.

A Businessman's Basic Shirt Collection

Fifteen shirts for business wear is a good *minimal, or starting, wardrobe*. No summer-weight cottons are included here, nor are the many weekend and casual wear shirts you will require as you expand your wardrobe.

5 white shirts
    2 broadcloth, 2 oxford cloth, 1 pinpoint oxford cloth
6 blue shirts
    2 oxford cloth, 1 pinpoint oxford cloth, 1 end-on-end, 2 striped
1 Bengal or other bold stripe
1 cream or ivory shirt (not tan or beige)
1 red and white stripe (or solid pink)
1 gray on white stripe

By the time he attains upper-level status, a manager's shirt wardrobe should contain nearly double the number of shirts outlined above, as follows:

9 white shirts
    3 broadcloth, 2 oxford cloth, 2 pinpoint oxford cloth, 1 Sea Island
        cotton, plus 1 formal white dress shirt
10 blue shirts
    1 oxford cloth, 3 pinpoint oxford cloth, 2 end-on-end, 3 striped, 1
        fine hairline stripe
2 Bengal or other bold stripe
2 cream or ivory
1 pale yellow
1 pink

1 red and white stripe

1 gray on white stripe

1 tattersall (an overall pattern: thin lines of two or more colors forming small squares)

You realize, I'm sure, that this guide is not gospel. It is a suggestion based on what I have observed to be top executives' norms. Emphasize your own best colors. If yellow makes you look good, three or four shirts in various shades of yellow would not be excessive.

Your Necktie: A Clear Message

Your company retains a prestigious new law firm. They send a pair of associates to your office, and one is wearing a violet tie with a yellow gometric design on it. You hear less of what that lawyer is telling you, and see less of what he is showing you. What you can't get out of your mind is that purple tie. The poor guy will have a long way to go to overcome the impression he has made.

That's not a farfetched story. It happens all the time. And nearly always, in real life, it is *negative* impressions that cause reactions. You can wear a notably handsome new tie, perfectly coordinated with a sparkling striped shirt—the combination reinforcing your reputation for authority and taste—and although it won't win you a promotion or increase the size of your year-end bonus, you will continue to be respected and regarded as an important person. But the sad fellow in the unfortunate purple tie might suffer directly from his lapse in taste; senior partners in his firm may refuse to consider him when a partnership opens.

All of that because of a tie? Absolutely. If you believe anything in this book, believe that your fellow Americans read volumes about your character by glancing at your tie. They'll decide whether to give you time or brush you off; take you seriously or regard you as inconsequential; try to push you around or realize you're powerful; feel superior to your place in the social order or see you as one who belongs. All that—and more—in your tie.

It would be a serious mistake to underestimate the importance of this smallest item in a man's overall look. People may not remember what else you are wearing, yet they often remember your tie. That's because your tie is usually the brightest in color of all the clothes you are wearing, and it is worn in a focal position, close to your face. So it follows: If your tie is the one item that people will remember, it should be a good one.

The objective of the finest makers is to make a tie that is resilient, that will hold together for its life, and that will tie easily with the "dimple" centered under the knot.

—STANLEY MARCUS, chairman emeritus of Neiman-Marcus stores

One thing in favor of a polka-dot tie is that one more spot doesn't matter.

—ANCIENT WHEEZE IN THE MEN'S WEAR FIELD

A Tie's Gotta Have a Name

In my talks I always stress that a businessman shouldn't own a tie that doesn't have a name. A tie needs a real name, like foulard, paisley, pindot, stripe, or solid. It should not be a vague brownish orange tie with squiggles here and there, or a tie that has triangular designs in the middle.

Names almost always refer to a tie's pattern or texture. These are the most prominent ones, all acceptable for business wear:

• **Solid colors.** Can be made of fabrics ranging from the finest silks and linens, wool challis (a lightweight worsted, pronounced *shal'-ee*), on through square-ended knits of wool or cotton.

• **Foulards.** Smooth silk or silk-blend ties, with a small repeat pattern—usually printed, sometimes woven—in harmonizing colors.

• **Stripes.** Most often made of repp, a ribbed or corded silk fabric. Sometimes they are subtle; most often they bear bold regimental striped patterns. Regimentals have their origin in the distinctive stripes of various British military regiments, but those meanings have been lost at the jumbled tie counters of the world.

• **Polka dots.** The smallest and dressiest of these are called pindots.

· **Paisleys.** An overall pattern of teardrop shapes, less formal and more colorful than the "neats" or foulards. Paisleys have an Indian flavor, and are about as vivid as business protocol will allow.

· **Ancient madders.** Pure silk, dark backgrounds with a wonderful "hand" (feel), and a distinctive hazy film—like that on a Concord grape—on the fabric.

Several other categories of ties are sometimes worn by businessmen who have sufficient authority or a singular approach to style, and can carry it off. But I don't recommend that you try them. Among these questionable patterns are *club ties:* solid twill backgrounds on which used to be embroidered the insignia of one's private club, but which are now woven with small tennis rackets, marlins, golf tees, or maybe an H or a Y from a university logo; *plaid ties:* even though some perfectly acceptable ones are made in light, summer-weight cottons or in wool for winter holiday wear, they are a bit too informal for the office; ties with *large polka dots:* any dot wider than one quarter of an inch.

Some patterns are completely unsuitable and should never be admitted to your tie rack. Among these are ties that tell a story or show a picture or have large gaudy symbols on them. A paisley is as colorful and frisky a tie as should be seen in an office. And no half-and-halfs—part foulard or neat pattern, part stripe. Remember, your tie must have a name, a clear one. The choices among the legitimately named ties are infinite. Stick with them.

Silk and Other Fabrics in Ties

Americans prefer to buy and wear silk neckties. Of nearly 100 million ties bought annually, Gerald Anderson of the Neckwear Association of America, Inc., told me, 41 percent are silk. Blends, including synthetics, cotton, wool, and linen, account for the balance.

The quality of fabric used by a tie manufacturer accounts for 60 percent of his costs. Unlike many other retail items. relatively little is spent for packaging and promotion. A better, higher-priced tie should mean it is made of finer, more expensive fabric. And the pattern is also a large part of the cost. Good designers do not come cheap. The colors and intricate patterns in ties by Hermès, Ralph Lauren, and J. G. Hook add significantly to their cost.

Some of the best silks are heavy. But among the finest silks that make the best knots you will also find lightweight fabrics. Isn't that a contradiction? Seemingly so. However, part of the answer lies in the *interlining*. Ties retain their shapes and their resilience thanks to a strip of canvas sewn inside them. Without it, they would show permanent wrinkles after being knotted and untied just three or four times. With lightweight silks, a heavier canvas is used; conversely, thinner, lighter canvas is used with heavier tie fabrics. Since you cannot see inside the tie, you need not be concerned with that old tale about the number of lines woven into the canvas being an indicator of its quality. But it is worth knowing that whether light or heavy, silks can be constructed into ties that will hold up through months and years of wear.

Steer clear of a tie if the label identifies it as having a polyester content. If blended with silk, polyesters offer extended wear, but who needs extra wear in a tie? Ties don't wear out. They have accidents. They become boring, and may need early retirement; but they don't need their lives extended.

The difference in cost between a silk tie and a silk/polyester blend is insignificant: $5–$15 in the overall cost of your outfit. So go for the best—go for silk.

By and large, your tie wardrobe will be chiefly silk, with a sprinkling of wool challis and a number of cotton summer ties. Linen ties are a temptation. They are beautiful, with a rich, luxurious look that just can't

Frank Lloyd Wright's often-quoted maxim is, "Observe the terminals; they are most important."

The terminals in clothes are jacket lapels and sleeve edges; trouser cuffs; collars and cuffs of shirts; and *ties*. All of these endings determine whether clothes fit the wearer and reflect current style. After years of narrowing and widening, suit coat lapels have settled at a 3½-inch width, and ties are at a reasonable width of 3¼ to 3½ inches (measured at the widest point).

be duplicated. But they wrinkle terribly, and require that you tie them skillfully or the old-knot creases will show.

The Right Size, the Right Knot

The pendulum of fashion persuades the overly style-conscious to vary their tie widths radically. But in the executive suites, ties remain a relatively constant 3¼ inches wide.

The length of ties, when tied, is also constant. The tip should extend down to the belt. Not below it. Nor above it. Ties are manufactured in lengths that range from 54 to 57 inches. The adjustment for the right length when tied, of course, comes from the balance between the ends before you tie the knot.

Consistency in lengths does not seem to be a high priority in the necktie industry. If you're tall, those three inches can make a difference. If you require a longer tie, don't confine yourself to the limited choice in a "tall-men's store." Try this method: When shopping for a tie, narrow your selection down to a few best bets, lay them out on the counter, and see which are the longest. Your decision is easy.

The proper length of the back piece? It is immaterial, as no one sees it. Just concentrate on having the front piece fall at your belt line.

Your collar shape and size largely determine the kind of knot you'll tie. A standard collar, one with a tab or pin or a button-down—all are best with a four-in-hand knot. That's the knot most conservative dressers have been tying all their lives. It particularly suits the newer, smaller collars. If

---

Right . . . Dress! And at Ease.

I always wondered why some men who otherwise dress well miss that one small detail—the tie-knot dimple. Then I learned that in the army they were not allowed that refinement in tying their khaki ties. Today it is not only permissible, it is nearly essential when dressing for excellence.

your technique includes Step 5, as shown in the diagram that follows, you're doing it right. If it doesn't, I urge you to include it. A dimple makes a difference. When it is missing, the effect is not quite polished.

TYING THE FOUR-IN-HAND KNOT

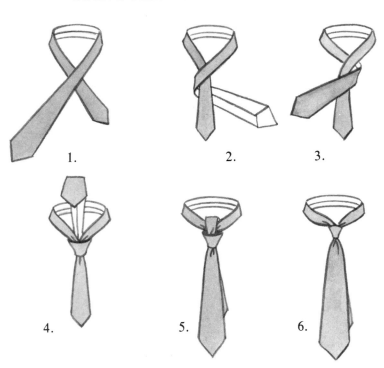

The four-in-hand is an elongated knot and is the most versatile and most often the appropriate one to wear.

1. Start with wide end of the tie extending a foot longer than the narrow end.
2. Cross wide end over narrow end, and back underneath.
3. Continue around, passing wide end across front of narrow end once more.
4. Pass wide end up through loop.
5. Holding front of knot loosely with index finger, pass wide end down through loop in front.
6. Remove finger and tighten knot carefully. While pulling down narrow end with one hand, use other hand to slide knot up snugly. Do not remove dimple; try to keep it as nearly centered as possible.

TYING THE HALF-WINDSOR KNOT

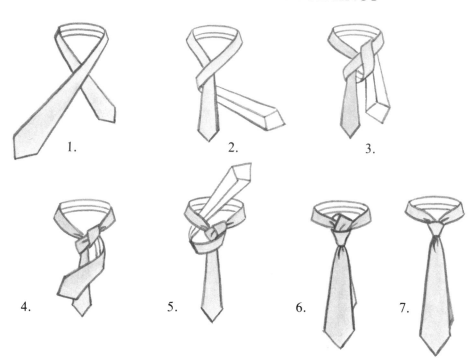

The half-Windsor is a more triangular and a slightly larger knot. It is proportioned for the shirt with a spread collar.

1. Start with wide end of tie extending a foot below narrow end. Cross wide end over narrow end.
2. Turn back underneath.
3. Bring up and turn down through loop.
4. Pass wide end around front.
5. Then up through loop.
6. And down through knot in front.
7. Tighten carefully and draw up snugly to collar.

Full Windsor knots are out of style and out of proportion for today's narrower ties. But if you like spread collars, the space between the points needs more knot that a four-in-hand provides. If you've ever seen a fellow with a skimpy knot lost in the gaping valley of a wide-spread collar, you know how strange it looks. Thus, the half-Windsor.

In a few years the pendulum might swing the other way. But for today and for several years to come, the four-in-hand is the knot you should be tying.

Which Tie for You?

Now we come to the core of the question, "What's the right tie to wear with the right shirt?" You've entitled to a straight answer—and on pages 126 to 128 you have a good part of it. Those pages contain charts that show specific color recommendations for specifically named colors of suits and shirts. *Those combinations will work*—I guarantee it.

Your selection process will be a little easier if you keep these tips in mind:

- Three master ties that are versatile and work where many other ties do not are a good, solid burgundy; a simple, widely spaced stripe, either a narrow blue line widely spaced on a red background or a narrow red line widely spaced on a blue background; and a *woven* pindot—not the usual *printed* pindot, but a tie in which the white dot is woven into navy blue fabric. This last is almost always an expensive tie, but it is worth the money.
- Arthur Klaus is recognized as one of the tie industry's authorities on design. He is executive vice-president for styling at Burma Bibas, a company that manufactures under the names of Oleg Cassini, J. G. Hook, and Londonderry. He says that red is currently the biggest seller in ties, with burgundy second. "Yellow is coming on very strong," Arthur says, "especially for the summer months. I see a trend toward slightly bolder pattern and colors in *fancies*." (Those are what the industry calls ties that don't fit into the classic categories.)
- Follow this basic rule: Your shirt should be lighter than your suit, and your tie should be darker than your shirt.

A Businessman's Basic Necktie Collection

18 to 20 silk ties
   3 solid colors—1 navy, 1 crimson, 1 burgundy—
   6 foulards—red, blue, burgundy, yellow backgrounds
   6 stripes—predominantly navy, red, burgundy, brown
   2 pindots—navy with white woven dots, blue with red dots
   1 club, only if it has important meaning for you

3 wool ties for more casual wear
   1 solid camel-colored
   1 solid knit—burgundy or dark blue
   1 patterned challis (possibly a paisley)

The Bow Tie Question

A general rule: You probably should not wear a bow tie to the office.

I tend to find bow tie wearers in academia (think of Arthur Schlesinger and George Will or your freshman-year English professor) or in professions requiring that people bend over drawing boards (they need a tie that won't get in the way). Sometimes, however, the guy in the bow tie is a very successful marketer or lawyer who merely prefers the flair and unconventionality of a bow tie. If that's you, and you have enough self-confidence to carry it off, what can I say? Only that you might better save this mode of self-expression for the weekends.

Caring for Your Ties

Always untie a necktie; sliding the knot invariably injures the fabric. It might also help to wash your hands before untying. Everyday living—even reading a newspaper—leaves deposits on your fingers that will soil your favorite ties.

Of course, hang your ties on a rack—the thicker the dowel on which they hang, the less chance of creasing. Knit ties are exceptions; they should be rolled loosely and kept in a drawer.

Pressing a tie to remove wrinkles just doesn't work—that is, not for most people and most ties. You or someone you live with may be an expert with an iron and know exactly how to go about steaming it. The only method that works is not to touch the tie with the iron. Lightly pass a steam iron back and forth an inch or so *above* the fabric. But if you're like the great majority of men, don't try it. Instead, hang the tie on a wooden hanger in a steamy bathroom, and see if the wrinkles come out. With a wool tie, they probably will; with a silk one, maybe not.

The neighborhood cleaner is not equipped to deal with pressing or cleaning delicate tie fabrics. He can remove spots, but then he will press the tie so that ridges from the lining show through. For the most part, a tie that is soiled, spotted, or horribly wrinkled has had it. Assume that you have had your money's worth from it and put it out to pasture.

If the spot is a small one, however, there is a solution. It is a cleaning compound that comes in an aerosol can. Goddard's Dry Clean is the name, and it is the only one I know that is worth using. It is sold in some men's clothing stores, hotels' sundries shops, and better hardware shops. I carry a small can on my travels. When a speck of gravy drops on your tie or suit, don't use club soda or any of those other alleged remedies. They only make matters worse. Let the spot dry. Later, spray on the Goddard's. If you follow precisely the directions on the can, the product *does* work.

Tie Crafters, a shop in New York City, has been in business for decades, cleaning ties and even narrowing them when fashions change. You can deal with them through the mail. Drop them a note at 116 East 27th Street, New York, NY 10016, or call (212) 867-7676. They will respond with a brochure that describes their services and charges. Another company will cut down oversize collars, shorten sleeves, replace worn collars and cuffs, and in general are stupendous shirt surgeons. Contact L. Allmeier, 19 West 23rd Street, New York, NY 10011, (212) 243-7390.

9

The Colors You Need in Your Wardrobe

Color Myths You Should Ignore

Color is the dominant factor in style, in clothing selection, and in dressing for excellence. It is so important that it has its own mythology.

How many of these not-so-truisms have you heard taken seriously?

Myth 1: Gray is always an appropriate color for business wear; all men look good in gray suits. Gray is the most versatile of business suit colors. It offers high flexibility, and is suitable for dressing up in a dark pinstripe, or for a casual appearance in a medium gray flannel. Gray *is* appropriate, but if you have sallow coloring—dark hair and olive-toned skin—gray can be unflattering. If you wear a gray suit, you must get heightened sparkle from your shirt and tie. Coordinate a gray suit with attractive colors: a red-and-white-striped shirt or yellow foulard tie, for instance.

Myth 2: Some men cannot wear blue suits. Almost every man can wear a navy suit and look distinguished. A dark blue suit is as much a part of the well-dressed businessman's wardrobe as is a dressy white shirt. For the few men who feel they don't look their best in a navy suit, there is some shade of dark blue that will work. A wardrobe can be assembled without a tan suit, without a glen plaid or a pinstripe; but no executive's wardrobe is complete without a dark blue suit.

Myth 3: Never wear blue and brown together. Definitely not true. Combinations of blue and brown can be extremely handsome and, in fact, are one of the "affluent looks." It is *dark* blue and *dark* brown that don't go together. But a navy blue blazer is compatible with every *light* shade of brown from winter white (the very palest brown) through beige, tan, camel, and khaki; all work wonderfully as sophisticated casual dress. And the reverse is also true: A camel-hair blazer worn with navy slacks is an equally smart look.

Myth 4: Men with light coloring should emphasize dark browns as their principal suit and coat colors. Despite the fact that men who have golden brown hair, or hazel or green eyes, or beige or peach-colored complexions do look good in dark brown, this color is not accepted in top business circles. Although chocolate or charcoal browns may be flattering to an executive's coloring, they should be worn only in tweeds and in casual attire.

Myth 5: For color and flair, a businessman can wear a wide range of pastel dress shirts: lavender, mauve, periwinkle blue, mint green, or peach. What is true is that these colors are often flattering, and they do work well in sportswear. But they are not for serious business wear; they do not reflect power or authority. These colors might make a wonderful statement in your summer necktie collection, but they should not be in evidence in the shirts you wear to work.

Myth 6: Redheads should never wear red. Depending on your shade of hair, there are a few tones of red that make fine necktie choices. With auburn hair, brick colors work well. Traffic-light reds are wrong. If your complexion is ruddy, you'd do well to keep away from red neckties altogether, since they impart a flushed, inflamed look.

Myth 7: Navy shoes may be worn with navy suits. Navy blue shoes carry a less than sophisticated connotation. With a navy suit, wear black shoes. You can bend this rule slightly and wear fine cordovans with navy suits, but black shoes are always a safe choice. (Navy socks are always appropriate with a blue suit. They are fully as acceptable with your black shoes as are black socks.)

Color Sends Power Messages

Two men went into one of the better stores in their city. They each bought a suit for $400, a good shirt, and a fairly expensive tie. When one wore his outfit to the office, he received compliments everywhere he turned. The other's outfit was never even noticed.

The punch line? The first man's three pieces were extremely well color-coordinated. They had verve. He chose each as a component of a single plan. (I will show you several never-fail versions of that plan—they're the easiest things in the world to follow.) The other man spent the same amount of money, but the clothes he bought had no connection with each other. A second-rate appearance was what he accomplished.

Color is free. Using it well costs no more than using it poorly.

Color can say a variety of things about you, depending on the kind of image you want to convey. Show up at an industrywide meeting in a dark blue, traditionally cut suit and everyone who looks at you is reassured. "He's okay. He's one of us." You're accepted; you belong.

If that suit were very dark blue, almost midnight blue, you might cause a little anxiety in some of your peers. The message they would get is, "This guy is a shade too elegant for this work session. Why is he so dressy? If he's that ambitious, perhaps we'd better watch out for him."

If the same suit were a lighter, medium blue, you might look like a casual middle-of-the-roader, and that's the niche they would put you in. An overly bright shade of blue, even slightly so, is downright incorrect. It will peg you as somewhere between the night manager of a suburban movie house and a messenger boy.

All this concluded from the color of a suit? I assure you it is. And it is done every day. That is why color is so important. Color in the business world is a subtle traditional power game and is best played according to established, traditional rules. It is perhaps the least understood element in dress. And it is the one that can make *the most* difference.

Knowing the color guidelines gives you freedom to move within them. First you have to know the rules. Then you can break them.

An invariable indicator of the appropriateness of a color: Darker is more formal; lighter is more casual. "Black tie" clothes, the ultimate in formality, are jet black. Summer weekend clothes might be cream color or white. Daytime business wear is most traditional when it is dark blue or dark gray.

A concern sometimes expressed to me about color is, "Won't I look drab, wearing a dark gray suit in a room filled with other dark gray shadows?"

I usually am able to lay that fear to rest. The questioner becomes involved with the possibilities of highlighting his own best colors, devising slight twists on classic color combinations, adding flair and verve to combinations of color and pattern.

Dressing as other executives do is not the hazard. *Looking unprofessional is.* You have my guarantee that after reading the next few pages, you will have left those hazards well behind you.

Three, and Only Three, Colors

There are three acceptable colors for men's business suits: blue, gray, and tan. Yet within those seemingly rigid confines you are offered choices of many shades and tones. Think about the variety of blue suits on the racks of a well-stocked store: darkest navy, almost indistinguishable from

Blue

George Washington is pictured almost exclusively in dark blue. And a psychologist (H. J. Eysenck) who tested more than 20,000 subjects found blue to be overwhelmingly their favorite color. With those precedents, there seems little risk that you will encounter anyone in the business world opposed to your blue suit, shirt, or tie.

black, solid or with a shadow stripe; slightly lighter blues, yet still very dark; medium blues, inclining toward either true or muted tones; lighter blue summer-weight suits, sometimes with a faint gray cast to their appearance. Every one of them is in the color family we call blue.

Gray suits range from the lightest, sometimes as a background for black and gray glen plaid weaves, to medium gray, on through deeper shades to banker's gray, charcoal, and even almost black. Browns range from off-white through beige, tan, khaki, camel, and medium brown up to dark chocolate brown.

Colors to Avoid

Cross the last color I mentioned from your list. As I've stated, dark browns are inappropriate in business wear. Among the top executives who retain my services, there is a strong feeling against solid brown suits. Harold Macmillan, former prime minister of England, observed that "gentlemen don't wear brown suits." Not everyone is affected that strongly. Some top men do wear especially fine dark brown suits and make them work. But other than in tweeds or plaids, it is usually safer to steer away from them. In contrast, tan, particularly in summer-weight clothes, is one of the classics.

Another color to avoid in business suits is very light gray. It is simply not worn in executive suites. Noncolors—hybrids that are dependent on "ish" for their existence—should also be avoided. Among them are brownish green, purplish blue, yellowish beige, and other lapses of designers' taste.

The Three-Color Rule: Within the three colors appropriate for business suits—blue, gray, and tan—the blues and grays should range from medium to dark; the tans should range from light to medium.

How to Determine
Your Own Best Color

In our society it is not considered good form to say to our friends, "Don't I have beautiful blue eyes?" But we can arrange it so that others notice our best features by our own wise choices.

A few months ago I was having lunch in one of New York's well-known restaurants, Sardi's. At a table nearby were three people. One of them was Paul Newman. He was dressed ultracasually in a crew-neck sweater, khaki pants, and an oxford cloth shirt. I noticed that the sweater was a shade of beige that exactly matched his sandy-colored hair. And the small bit of shirt that showed above the sweater was the very same blue as his remarkable eyes. His clothes made him look terrific. And *he* doesn't need much help!

How do you determine your own best colors? Certainly there is more to it than simply matching or contrasting your hair and eyes. Learn to trust your mirror. On some days, after getting dressed in the morning, you may look in the mirror and say to yourself, "Wow! I look pretty good today." And we all know those other days when you see your reflection and ask yourself, "Could I possibly look that bad?" It's almost always a matter of color. Certain colors and specific shades of those colors near the face do great things for you. Remember which shades made you look your best and wear them often.

Occasionally other people will tell you. When you receive two or more *unsolicited* compliments on your dress, you know that something you are wearing is a good color for you. If, on the other hand, you come to the office in what you feel is a well-pulled-together outfit and people ask, "Were you up late last night?," you probably are wearing the wrong colors.

According to Sandra Merrill Herscott, who teaches color at the Boston Architectural Center in Boston, "Color is a form of energy. If the color you are wearing is correct for you, all of a sudden there is a burst of energy. Your eyes light up and look clearer. You look dynamic, with a healthy glow. This causes other people to respond to you by having a longer attention span and being more receptive. They are more comfortable with you. If you wear wrong colors, you look older, tired, and lose your individuality. Your skin can turn sallow, you get circles under the eyes and shadows around the mouth—giving you the look of a five-o'clock shadow early in the morning."

Your Natural Color, Plus . . .

Let's consider some of the ways you can match colors to flatter your skin and hair tones. *Do you have dark, Mediterranean coloring? Black or dark brown hair, dark eyes, and an olive skin?* You want to apply the *opposite* of Newman's strategy: Instead of repeating dark colors, which will create a drab, depressing effect, you should *contrast* your coloring. Steer clear of dark browns, mustards, khakis, and olive drabs. You need light, crisp, clear colors. Wear shirts that are white, light blue, pink, cream, pale yellow, or the cleanest and lightest of grays. With them you can wear ties in deep, vivid tones of red, blue, or yellow, and patterned mixtures of any harmonizing colors. Your shirt and tie will frame your face. They will act as a foil, giving needed contrast to your skin coloring and allowing you to wear the traditional dark grays and blues in suit colors that announce your membership among the insiders.

If you are black, you may be able to wear a wide range of colors, but usually your coloring works best with colors that favor a dark, Mediterranean cast. With my dark hair and olive skin, I have always said, "I look good in any color as long as it is white or powder blue." One reason that white and light blue are the classic colors for men's shirts is that they flatter the broadest range of people.

But suppose your complexion is not dark. *Suppose you are very fair, with blond hair and light blue eyes*—they called you a "towhead" when you were little. Wearing pale colors can give you a washed-out, flat appearance. You want variations. The basic theme builds in contrast: a dark suit, white or light blue shirt or any assertively striped shirt (red and white, burgundy and white, dark blue and white, even green and white), and a tie that is darker than the shirt. In the summer, if you are tanned, you can choose combinations from the lighter end of the palette. Your skin will have created the contrast that is necessary for dash and definition in an outfit.

Rule: Accent your eye or hair color if it is light. Contrast your eye, hair, and complexion coloring if it is dark.

If your hair is gray, there is nothing but clear sailing ahead, from an image standpoint. You have the physical requisites of that often-mentioned "command presence," and adding the clothing components is fairly easy. Add pink to your wardrobe of shirts. With gray hair and a gray suit, a crisp white shirt can project an image that is flintlike and cold. Sometimes that's useful. But a pink or red-and-white-striped shirt adds warmth and vitality—it is very flattering. By the time a man is old enough to have gray hair, he should be sure enough of his masculinity to be comfortable wearing pink. A pink shirt is an excellent addition to any shirt wardrobe. When I talk on college campuses, my remarks about pink shirts are occasionally greeted with snickers. But most young men, especially in eastern seaboard schools, find pink shirts as much a part of their Ivy League uniform as khaki pants.

Color Combinations:
Formulas for Success

Color coordinating your clothes serves two purposes. One is to make you look good; the other is to help you look organized and professional. A matched look makes a positive, nonverbal statement about you.

Here's the key to it all. . . .

Start with your suit. It is gray, blue, or tan. If gray or blue, it's best to stay with the darker shades. Whichever you select, it should be clearly one color; that is, avoid blue-gray. Double colors make suits impossible to match with ties and shirts. Buy a suit that is a true blue or gray—with no trace of a second color—and you will find it much easier to coordinate the colors of your shirt and tie.

Let's say your suit is dark gray. Choose a light-colored shirt. Nothing is lighter than white, and white is never wrong. It is always elegant. But you'd like a little dash in your appearance today, so you pick a pale yellow shirt, a cotton broadcloth with a pin collar. You're exactly on target. The one essential rule of color coordination is falling into place: **Your shirt should be lighter than your suit; your tie should be darker than your shirt.** All you need now is to go to your tie rack, and select one that blends together the gray and yellow. It might be a paisley or foulard, a black background with yellow highlights. It might be a silk tie, diagonally striped, with black or gold as one of the dominant colors.

Everything else—important suggestions and variations and assorted tips—that you will want to know about color coordination follows easily from this rule. **Another rule: The lighter the shirt and the darker the suit and tie, the more formal the look.**

The gradations of light/dark dressing are fascinating. They are logical as well. Let me show you what I mean. "Black tie" is the ultimate in light/dark dressing: darkest of dark suits, whitest of white shirts, and an appropriate black tie to round it off. You can't get much more formal than that. (Chapter 10 features three detailed charts to show you the "for-

Gray Is Grand

A gray suit can take you everywhere. It is dressy enough for situations where you must be assertive, but not too overpowering for less formal occasions.

Gray suits are the backbone of a businessman's wardrobe. He cannot have too many of them or too many different types. When a crucial meeting is in the offing, and he's not sure just what to wear, he can safely reach into his closet and select a gray suit. It is sure to be right.

A gray suit wardrobe *could* include two very dark charcoal gray suits, both solid, but one a winter flannel and one a lighter-weight ten-month suit; a very dark gray pinstripe; two dark gray shadow stripes, one winter- and one summer-weight; a dark gray tick weave or mini-herringbone weave, or both; a medium gray hard-finished worsted; a double-breasted gray and white glen plaid on the dapper, dressy side; another medium gray single-breasted glen plaid with a fine blue line in the pattern; and a medium gray go-anywhere suit.

Obviously this is not a typical wardrobe. But a man who dresses superbly could find a reason to own any or all of these gray suits and might even find himself in a clothing store looking for another gray suit.

Gray goes marvelously well with most colors: green, yellow, maroon, all shades of blue. Avoid wearing gray ties with gray suits. Since grays have many undertones of green and other colors, two different grays almost never work together. But gray with almost anything else is a winner!

mality ratios" of nearly every color and pattern of suit, shirt, and tie.) Moving down the scale of formality to the most dressy daytime business wear, you might wear a navy pinstripe suit, a white shirt, and a dark blue tie with white or gray pindots. Moving still further away from formality, you might have a medium-dark blue suit, blue-and-white-striped shirt, and a red tie. As you darken the color of the shirt and lighten the color of the tie, the outfit becomes more casual.

Several years ago, when Jimmy Carter was in the White House, he invited Egyptian President Anwar Sadat and Israeli Prime Minister Menachem Begin to come to the United States. He arranged for them to meet at Camp David to negotiate an agreement. All of the official photos that came out of the Camp David meetings showed Begin and Sadat dressed in almost identical versions of the diplomatic look—dark blue pin-striped suits, starched white shirts, and the most formal and elegant of navy blue ties with small white pindots. President Carter was always pictured in much more informal business attire—a medium blue suit, light blue shirt, and burgundy tie. His choice of clothes was no accident. They were carefully selected to show that he was not part of the actual negotiations, but only the host.

The 1-2-3 of Color

Wearing **two colors** is the top executives' conventional way of dressing. It is expected; it is always correct and it never goes out of style. Also, it is the most striking. If you are walking down the street and notice someone who is exceptionally well dressed, you may turn around to see what he has done to catch your eye. Almost always he will be wearing only two colors. A navy suit, blue shirt, and burgundy and blue tie is an often-seen, supersafe example.

Two-color dressing is safe and easy. It offers possibilities for dozens and dozens of elegant combinations. I recommend it because once you have the hang of it, you can practically never go wrong. It becomes second nature.

- Start with the suit. It is your base color.
- Add a second, contrast color with the shirt. It is your accent.
- With the tie you *tie* it all together by repeating the two colors.

Your suit, let's say, is dark gray, making gray your base color. Next you add a shirt in a contrasting light color, perhaps a red and white fine hairline stripe. Now you have two colors—gray and red. (The white in a striped shirt doesn't count.) Your third selection is the necktie. Since what you want to do is tie the color combination together, you choose a red or burgundy foulard tie with a small gray pattern. Your three-piece outfit is complete and you have stayed with two colors.

The trick to pulling off **one-color dressing** successfully is a practiced eye at discerning shades, and some interest in combining textures of fabric. (We'll explore the possibilities of working with *texture* and *pattern* in the next two chapters.) For the present, unless you are extremely skillful, one-color dressing may look dull. Or, worse, the shades of the color may clash, as with a periwinkle tie worn with a navy pinstripe suit.

Yet I do see variations. Very often extremely successful men who project a sophisticated, well-traveled image dress in one color (actually, in various shades of one color family): a gray suit, white shirt, and predominantly black tie with a silver pattern. Or a blue and white glen plaid suit, pale blue shirt, and navy tie with white dots. Or a tan poplin summer suit, cream-color broadcloth shirt, and a brown and off-white tie. All of these outfits are one-color dressing. And all display the authority of a dynamic, knows-his-own-mind achiever.

Shirt/Tie Color Combinations That Work

Some morning when you are dressing you may put together an outfit that your mirror tells you doesn't quite make it. If you're not exactly sure what is wrong, check to see how many colors you are wearing. Generally you will have added a heavy dose of an extra color. I don't mean that you can't have a third color in a stripe or in the small pattern in your tie, but basically your eye should see two colors. It's easy to correct the not-quite-perfect outfit simply by changing your tie. Put on one that combines the colors in your suit and shirt, once again proving that color is free. You needn't always buy new clothes. Often it only takes choosing the right item from your closet.

One automotive executive at a seminar in Las Vegas protested: "You tell us to use restraint in choosing shirt colors—the lightest, softest pale blues and ivories. And then you tell us to try for dash and flair. Which is it?"

I do advocate both those approaches. Yet it isn't hedging. It is further proof of the versatility of color combinations, all perfectly acceptable as long as none of the taste taboos is violated.

Solid-color shirts are eminently right for all occasions. And yes, they should be pale tones. Dark solid colors—heavy shades of purple, orange, green, or brown—simply have no place in a businessman's wardrobe.

Yet smart combinations can be built around a striped shirt—fairly assertive stripes of red, blue, green, brown, or gray on a white background. Once again, the light/dark rule comes into play. On a gray-and-white-striped shirt, which becomes paler when seen from across a room, you want to wear a tie dark enough to dominate it. A neat pearl gray pattern on a dark red field is a handsome choice.

Two colors which are currently enjoying popularity as strong accents in neckties are yellow and red. A small-patterned foulard with a yellow background can be a dashing look on either a white shirt or a blue shirt. This is one of those instances where the color combination does not really fit the rules—it just looks great.

But nothing is more popular today than the red tie. It comes in every variation of color and appears in every one of the accepted patterns, from the most formal pindot to the most casual paisley. You see it in all textures from an elegant silk to a wool knit. It's hard to go wrong with a red tie.

Active Self-Confidence

Red affects all people in the same way, no matter how old they are or what culture they live in. It's always exciting, stimulating, activating. It expresses vital force and self-confidence.

—DR. MAX LUSCHER,
The 4-Color Person
(Simon and Schuster, 1977)

Blue-and-white-striped shirts have a whole hierarchy of their own. A hairline stripe, the thinnest of pale blue lines woven into cotton fabric, is one of the more elegant looks for business wear. You won't find it in every store, but there is generally a good representation of this aristocrat of shirts in finer shops. A wider stripe of blue, particularly on oxford cloth, is rather preppy. However, it is a classic and totally acceptable if you are wearing a natural-shouldered suit. (I have always found striped, button-down oxford shirts discordant—somehow wrong in "spirit"—when worn with a padded-shoulder, more formally cut suit.)

The possibilities of wider spacings and stronger shades of blue stripes are challenging. They are harder to coordinate with suits and ties, yet can be highly effective. You'd do well to postpone experimenting with them until you have the basics down pat.

In replying to the automotive executive's question, I'd have to stress that subtle differences in color make strong differences in image. Pale blue, when crisp and in top condition, is among the most elegant of colors. When lacking luster or when it is a blue-gray color, it appears faded and washed out. The message it sends is "old, low quality, cheap."

A shirt in powder blue, that most versatile hue, can be wonderful in the right combinations for year-round business, social, and casual wear. But some powder blues are slightly on the greenish blue side. They are practically impossible to coordinate. Others have the slightest hint of

---

All Hit, No Miss

How do you go about putting together a color-coordinated outfit? There is one, and only one, way to make certain you are buying exactly the right tone of cream at the shirt counter, that the paisley tie you're buying doesn't have a green with too much yellow in it and that they work together. The secret is to *match them up right there in the store before you pay for them.*

When your new suit is being marked for alterations, tell the fitter to save a scrap from the pants leg. He will be glad to give it to you. Often he can cut a small piece for you to take with you right then. Take the piece with you when buying shirts and ties for that suit. Or better still, wear the suit itself on your shirt and tie buying trip. Always buy the shirts and ties together, as coordinated purchases.

If you trust to your memory of exactly what shade, out of literally hundreds, you're trying to match, you've got three elements that might go wrong: your memory, your judgment, and the salesman's perception of what color you are describing. By removing any question of memory from the process and improving your judgment, color coordination will cease to be a problem.

purple. If you are good with color, you can pull off a wonderful combination by wearing one of these with just the right blue and red tie. From a slight distance, your tie will assume a faint purple cast that blends beautifully with that shade of powder blue. Isn't it odd that a fine-quality tie in blue and red that gives a cast of purple works wonderfully while a purple tie puts you down as a tasteless dresser?

Repeating Colors in Your Accessories

Coordinating the three basic elements—your suit, tie, and shirt—has ensured that two of the three will be in the same color family, or that they will be close cousins. Having established that basic color, you will want to repeat it and to be sure that none of your accessories clash with it. Among them are:

· **Shoes.** Wear black with a blue or gray suit, dark brown with tan suits: easy and obvious and, once again, correct.

One of the most frequently asked questions at my seminars is, "What color shoes do I wear with the weekend combination of navy blazer and khaki trousers?" My answer is, "Cordovan, the third color for a basic shoe wardrobe." This is a dark brown with a good deal of red in it, although not as red as burgundy. A cordovan shoe is one of the classics. With increasing sophistication in your dressing skills, you can even wear cordovan shoes with gray suits. But that is part of the wonderfully subtle world of dressing in "neutrals," and not something you'd want to try tomorrow.

You may have noticed that I haven't mentioned white shoes. When I speak in the South, the one place where I have a few minutes of strain with my audience is when I say how I feel about white shoes!

White shoes are not part of executive dress—not in the South; not anywhere. It is true that men do wear white shoes in all parts of the country, but nowhere do really well-dressed top managers wear white shoes. Oh, yes, they wear them on the tennis courts, sometimes for weekends when they decide to go collegiate and wear white bucks, and even occasionally they can be acceptable on the golf course. That is where it stops. Many not-so-knowledgeable men do wear them. But never will you see a president of a large company lunching in a fine club or attending a stockholders' meeting wearing white shoes. The same goes for white leather belts. They are taboo.

No doubt your next question is, "Well, if I should not wear white shoes even on weekends, what do I wear with white trousers?" The answer is dark shoes and dark socks. When you are not used to it, it may seem strange. But the next time you see a man of the type who might be on an international list of well-dressed men and he is wearing white, cream, or light tan trousers, notice his shoes. They will be dark. He may not even be wearing a seemingly essential element of clothes—socks. For some reason, the style of not wearing any socks at all is extremely popular for weekend dressing. I am not referring to sports clothes and casual dress. I'm referring to the Palm Beach look of a slubbed silk tweed sportscoat, a fine cotton shirt worn with a tie or open at the neck, lightweight wool gabardine trousers, highly polished Gucci loafers, and *no socks*.

    · **Socks.** With tan or khaki suits and dark brown shoes, wear dark brown socks. With gray suits and black shoes, wear charcoal gray or black socks. With blue suits and black shoes, wear either navy blue or black socks. The code of dress for executives is quite rigid about the color of footwear: *Socks are always darker than the pants.* Black socks are darkest of all, and therefore always safe.

    · **Belt.** Repeat the shoe color—brown or black.

    · **Suspenders.** If worn instead of a belt, suspenders should coordinate with the shirt or tie color.

    · **Pocket square.** Wearing it at all is optional. If you do choose one, echo rather than accurately repeat the color and pattern of your tie. Matching sets of foulard ties and pocket squares are out. Reds and yellows as the dominant colors in ties are so strong that you would probably not want to repeat them in a pocket square. I notice the trend, led by impeccably tailored men, back to white linen handkerchiefs in breast pockets. And only a small casual bit showing is a surer bet than the precisely peaked four tips of yesterday.

That One in Every Eleven

If you are the one in every eleven men who is color-blind, you will find it next to impossible to select the tones and shades necessary for exact harmony. If your ability to differentiate between shades is less acute than it might be, here is a tested, foolproof solution.

Ask a friend who has good taste and is not color-blind to spend an hour or so with you, going through your entire collection of suits, shirts, ties, and socks. Arrange the clothing into compatible combinations, following the guidelines in this chapter. On the label of each piece, use an indelible marker to identify its set by number. For example, all shirts and ties that coordinate with gray suit #3 are marked "#3." A trick that works with socks: Buy all your black ones from one manufacturer and all your brown ones from another, choosing brands that have some identifiable stitching on the toe. And, of course, ask that same friend with the good eye for color to come along when you are buying new clothing.

As so many men are color-blind, it makes little sense to be embarrassed or hide the fact from the salesman when shopping for clothes. He sees people who are color-blind every day. Ask him, for example, to show you a blue shirt with no green or purple in it. (That can be helpful even if you are not color-blind.)

Factual, Actual Combinations for Business Wear

It's one thing to know the Dow-Jones Theory; it's another to name four stocks that will go up 50 percent by the end of the year. It's the same with the principles of color coordination. What you require, right now, are some inside tips for putting the rules you have learned into practice and knowing exactly which color shirt and tie to wear with which color suit.

Mathematically, the three charts I have included here will yield hundreds of combinations. Yet they have been reduced to a minimal number of factors. That way, they are easy to use as a day-to-day guide, one that you will find practical until you get the hang of combining elements on your own.

Keep in mind that *all shirts listed here are plain or striped*. For business wear, checked or plaid patterns are rarely acceptable. If you do see an unobtrusive check that you simply must buy, it's safest to wear a solid-color tie with it for weekend blazer dressing.

The only plaid suit regarded as acceptable in the business world is that marvelously subtle pattern the glen plaid. It is a useful suit for every man's wardrobe—less formal than a navy pinstripe, more interesting than a solid color. In Europe sophisticated men know this pattern as Prince des Galles, or Prince of Wales. Even so, I'd advise you not to invest in

WHEN YOUR SUIT IS BLUE . . .

Ranging from dark blue to navy so intense it might almost be mistaken for black, dark blue suits are synonymous with power. They are worn by the CEOs of the nation's largest banks and the CEO of the nation itself. Available in solids, pinstripes, and luxurious tick weaves, every business wardrobe is topped with the suits that say assertively, "I mean business."

DARK BLUE SUIT—SOLID SHADE

Shirt*	Solid or Dominant Color of Tie	Secondary Color (if patterned tie)
white	red	blue, white, or yellow
	blue	red, white, or yellow
	yellow	blue or red
light blue (or blue stripes)	navy	red, white, or cream
	red	blue, cream, or white
	yellow	blue or red
yellow	navy	blue or yellow
	blue	yellow or red
pink (or red stripes)	blue	white or red
	burgundy	blue or white
	yellow	burgundy
cream	blue	cream, red, or white
	burgundy	cream, blue, or white

*When wearing a striped shirt, the third column becomes especially important. Your tie selection is trickier, so spend a little more time selecting the right one.

BLUE SUIT—PATTERNED

Suit	Plain Shirt	Tie Colors—Solid or Dominant Color If Patterned
glen plaid, red lines	white	blue or red
	blue	navy or claret
	pink	burgundy
glen plaid, rust lines	white	blue or rust
	blue	rust
pinstripe, gray lines	white	red, blue, or yellow
	blue	red, blue, or yellow
	pink	burgundy
pinstripe, white lines	white	red, blue, or claret
	blue	red, blue, or claret
	pink	burgundy

Navy blazers are not worn to most offices. But if your company's dress code permits, use this guide: Let the trouser color you select determine your choice of shirt:

Gray or khaki trousers—pink, white, blue, or yellow shirt and tie

White trousers—pink, blue, or yellow shirt

WHEN YOUR SUIT IS GRAY . . .

"He's authoritative, serious, has the capacity to take charge. And yet he's not pushing. He has assurance." A dark gray suit can say all that about its wearer. And who wouldn't want to give that impression as he walks into a room? The range of shades, from smoke on through charcoal, is wide enough to accommodate any taste. As base colors for glen plaids, stripes—chalk, red, or blue lines are handsome and eminently proper—and tick weaves, grays are the most adaptable colors in your suit closet.

GRAY SUIT—SOLID SHADE

Shirt	Solid or Dominant Color of Tie	Secondary Color (if patterned tie)
white	red	yellow, black, or green
	dark green	black, red, or yellow
	black	yellow, red, or blue
	yellow	red or blue
blue	blue	yellow, white, or green
	yellow	black, gray, or blue
	black	yellow, green, or blue
pale yellow	dark green	burgundy or ivory
	black	yellow
pink (or red stripes)	burgundy	black, blue, or gray
	black	red, yellow, or gray
pearl gray (or gray stripes)	red	black, yellow, blue, or gray
	black	red, blue, or gray
	yellow	black, red, or gray
cream	red	black, yellow, or blue
	black	red, blue, or gray
	yellow	black, red, or gray
	dark green	yellow, burgundy, or cream

GRAY SUIT—PATTERNED

Suit	Plain Shirt	Tie Colors—Solid or Dominant Color If Patterned
glen plaid or pinstripe, blue lines	white	black, yellow, or blue
	cream	black, red, or blue
	blue	burgundy
	pink	blue or burgundy
glen plaid or pinstripe, white lines	white	black, gray, red, or dark green
	light blue	black, gray, or blue
glen plaid or pinstripe, red lines	white	black, yellow, or red
	pearl gray	black, gray, or red

WHEN YOUR SUIT IS TAN . . .

No matter that solid dark browns are inadmissible as suit colors for a serious executive. Strike off that end of the range, and you are left with a gorgeous palette of summer tans, khakis, and olives. Darker browns emerge as adaptable backgrounds for glen plaids and—in academia and some industries—a wide variety of sportscoats.

TAN SUIT—SOLID SHADE

Shirt	Solid or Dominant Color of Tie	Secondary Color (if patterned tie)
white	tan	olive, yellow, or brown
	red (all shades)	tan, white, or yellow
	yellow	olive, brown, or red
blue	brown	olive, blue, or yellow
	blue	brown, khaki, or yellow
	yellow	brown, olive, or blue
yellow	red	yellow
	brown	olive, yellow, or green
	olive	green, gold, or brown
pink (or red stripes)	blue	yellow or red
	olive	yellow or red
cream	brown	green, blue, or off-white
	olive	green, gold, or blue
	green	brown, gold, or blue

TAN SUIT—PATTERNED

Suit	Plain Shirt	Tie Colors—Solid or Dominant Color If Patterned
glen plaid, blue lines	white	blue or tan
	blue	tan, brown, or blue
	cream	blue, gold, or tan
glen plaid, red lines	white	blue, red, or brown
	ivory	blue, red, yellow, or brown
tweed sportscoat (in this case, the coat can range from medium to dark brown)	white	brown, yellow, or blue
	blue	brown, green, or blue
	yellow	brown, green, or blue
	cream	brown, green, olive, or blue
	pink	brown, burgundy, or off-white

one until you have seen a glen plaid worn by more than one of the shakers and movers of your firm.

One reason many men steer away from plaids is that they are not sure exactly how to work with the pattern. The three charts of color combinations allow for glen plaids and specify "lines" of one color or another. Those are the fine, single lines of another color woven into the fabric. When buying a glen plaid suit, keep a watchful eye on the small line of color in the pattern. (If you are color-blind, ask the salesman, and then ask the tailor for confirmation.)

Although some extremely fine glen plaid suiting fabrics come without the extra color line, most come in muted shades of blue, gray, or brown with that fine line. This ever-so-subtle line is the one to check carefully. If it is red, rust, or blue, fine. They are excellent colors to use for accents. But if the fine line is mustard color or orange, as it often is, you could be forced into collecting mustard or orange ties—a somewhat alarming prospect.

On the other hand, a medium brown glen plaid often has a fine blue line in it, which makes for handsome combinations. You can wear a light blue shirt for your accent and then find a brown tie with a small blue pattern or a blue diagonal stripe. You will be dressed in two colors, perfectly coordinated and with a dash of originality.

Tan to One You'll Earn Compliments

A tan suit offers needed variation. It extends your color palette beyond the blues and grays.

It allows you to wear a *light* suit, which can be a welcome addition to an otherwise dark wardrobe of suits.

It works well with a *suntan,* and thus has its own built-in repetition of color.

Notice how logical men's styles are. Contrast is essential. In winter months when we are pale, dark suits are all that are appropriate. In summer, with a tan (or a bit of bronzer), light tan suits are added to the closet, giving you variation, repeating the color of your skin, and emphasizing your tan as well.

You will notice that the combination I just described combines blue and brown. Men often say, seeing the combinations of blue and brown that I show, "I have always heard that you are not supposed to wear blue and brown together." Not true. Actually brown and blue are a highly workable color combination.

Dark blue and *dark* brown do not work together. But tan and most shades of blue are great combinations. Examples are a navy suit, cream-color shirt, and navy and beige tie; a navy blazer with khaki-colored trousers; a camel-hair blazer with navy trousers; a medium brown glen plaid suit or brown tweed jacket and light blue shirt; a tan suit with a blue shirt and almost any shade of brown or blue in the tie.

10

Pattern:
The Silent Persuader

Add what you now know about *color* to an understanding of how *pattern* brings life and distinction to your appearance, and you have most of the basics of dressing for excellence. Pattern is the foundation for building your individual image.

Myths About Pattern You Can Ignore

Men's clothing, as we recognize it today, has evolved from styles that were set in the United States and England about seventy years ago. During those decades, several myths about the use of patterns also grew. Today, those in the know recognize that the beliefs are groundless.

Now is the time for you to abandon . . .

Myth 1: Never combine three solid colors; the result is bound to be dull. Want proof that this is untrue? Consider a dark blue suit, white shirt, and solid crimson tie: effortless polish. Or a tan gabardine suit, white shirt, and yellow tie. Or another flawless combination of three solids: medium gray suit, white shirt, and charcoal gray tie. Obviously three solid colors can be combined in highly interesting ways.

Myth 2: Wear only one patterned item of clothing; all others should be solids. Believe that and your appearance is sure to be dated, and about as lively as dishwater. Later in this chapter you will find detailed formulas and examples for combining two patterns when you choose a suit, shirt, and tie.

Myth 3: If wearing two patterns is good, wearing three ought to be better. Three patterns *can* be worn at once, most effectively, by sophisticated dressers. But whenever the question is asked, my advice is, "Never wear three patterns together unless you have impeccable taste—and you're not the only one who thinks so."

Now, leaving myth for reality, let's consider how you can most easily put patterns to work in your wardrobe.

The Look of the Feel

Patterns in men's clothes are either woven into the fabric or printed on it. The chalk stripe in a suit and the stripe in an oxford cloth shirt are woven into the material.

Some lightweight cloths—notably silk in ties—have the design printed on their surfaces. Whether woven or printed, the pattern (or design element) is usually flat. As with a painting, the visual impact comes from the placement and repetition of colors—stripes or dots, checks or bars, solid bands or swirling paisleys.

Yet there is another way to create pattern. More properly, it is the *illusion* of pattern. That is through texture, which is easily recognized when you lightly pass your fingers over a piece of flannel, say, as opposed to a piece of silk. What is interesting about *texture* as a pattern, or design element, is subtle. You don't have to touch it to know it's there: The play of light and shadow makes it visible, even when the entire garment is a single color. Wool gabardine and cotton twill suits, or a summer weekend jacket of shantung (irregularly weighted) silk, are examples: The look is in the "feel" of the goods. (You'll learn all the uses of texture in the next chapter.)

Putting Patterns Together

During the programs I present, I'm frequently interrupted with questions from men in the audience. More than any other topic, except perhaps the cost of clothing items, businessmen are concerned with *coordinating* their suits, shirts, and ties. Here are some of the more frequently asked questions. They may echo some of your own uncertainties about what is really an easy-to-acquire skill.

Q. I think I understand about color-coordinating my clothes. But now you toss in pattern. Won't that come in conflict with the color principles you just discussed?

A. Not at all. The color harmonies you're going to practice are a vital first step toward dressing for excellence. Now you will go a step further, using *pattern* to enhance and enliven the business wardrobe you have selected, making it more sophisticated.

Q. Why do "experts" keep saying don't mix patterns?

A. The answer isn't flattering. The books are written by people who think that American men can't learn to do it. I know for a fact that you *can*. It's really very easy to do. After all, if you can learn how to run a business, you can learn how to wear two patterns together. I'm going to show you how, and I guarantee you'll have no problem.

Q. Even though you say it's difficult to achieve, can you give me an example of three-pattern coordination?

A. A shadow-striped suit, with the stripe so faint you almost see the suit as a solid dark gray, a red-and-white-striped shirt, with the red so subtle that when seen eight feet away the shirt appears to be light pink, and a red foulard tie with a gray pattern, neat and small and tasteful.

You *can* wear three patterns together, but first let's learn how to manage two flawlessly.

Combining Two Patterns

Imagine a large, oversize drawing of a blue-and-white-striped shirt. The stripes are exaggeratedly wide and equidistant, for emphasis. I own such a drawing; it is a prop, made especially for use in my seminars.

On this striped shirt I place an overscaled solid dark blue tie. Everyone agrees that the tie is a correct and safe choice. But now consider another selection—a tie with navy background and close-together white polka dots. When I show this tie on the striped shirt, the audience groans.

What is wrong with this choice? It is not that polka dots can't go with stripes, but rather that the close-together dots seem to fight with the stripes. By replacing the many-dotted tie with another tie that has the same-sized dots but more widely spaced, the eyestrain and clashing sensation are relieved. The combination works.

The rule, when mixing two patterns: **Avoid combining two large, busy patterns. Combine one small pattern with one that is larger and more widely spaced.**

Now picture the next step—a red, green, and yellow paisley tie on the same blue-and-white-striped shirt. It looks terrible. The mistake is *not* that a paisley tie is all wrong with a striped shirt. (Although the exaggerated, horsey effect of my demonstration tie doesn't help matters. In real life, you would use a more subdued stripe in the shirt and a smaller, muted paisley pattern.) The problem is that the colors are dreadful together. The tie and shirt break the two-color rule with a vengeance, combining blue, red, green, and yellow.

When combining two patterns, you must **make certain that the colors are exceptionally well-coordinated.** The two patterns should not look as though they just happened to fall together, but rather that they were the result of thoughtful planning.

What kind of paisley would have pulled together that blue striped shirt and a dark blue or gray suit? One in which the two-color pattern was predominantly blue and that wonderful tone of creamy white you find in a rich, authentic paisley. Or, if the shirt were red-and-white-striped, the paisley pattern might have been gray, red, and black. Pattern and color work together. When they're wrong, they are destructive; when they are right, you look terrific—and gain high marks for being imaginative and creative as well.

"Formal to Casual" at a Glance

How great it would be if you had a clear, easy-to-use quick-reference guide, rating suits, shirts, and ties for their suitability to every kind of business and social wearing. Well, you do have that guide; it's in the form of three charts on the next few pages.

What a breakthrough! I designed the charts especially for this book. As far as I know, there is nothing like them anywhere. The three guides are related numerically (I'll explain that in a moment), giving you perfect-every-time coordination of the color, pattern, and style of your entire look.

As part of each chart, you'll find a set of notes and special tips: details that will help you be absolutely sure of the look you want to achieve.

Why and How the Charts Work

The easiest suit to coordinate into your wardrobe and one which will never lead you into appearance disasters is a solid dark one, either blue or gray. A smooth-finished worsted is a good choice, so there is no texture to be considered, either.

But life offers you more than forever playing it safe. That's where the first chart, "Suit Patterns, Formal to Casual," enters the picture. I know you can handle all twenty-one of the pattern possibilities on it. Starting with number 1, the "white tie and tails" that Fred invariably wore when stepping out with Ginger, the chart proceeds through various degrees of formality—all the way through to the most casual of casual wear: sports clothes with jeans or shorts.

Do not overlook the fact that numbers *4 through 11,* and only those numbers, are suitable for most business wear. Numbers *12 through 15* are for more casual industries and for academia. Some West Coast companies and glamour industries might even include *16 through 18* within the range of what is appropriate.

[TEXT CONTINUES ON PAGE 142]

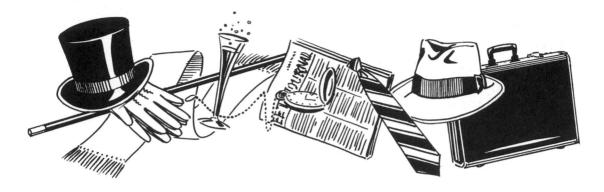

SUIT PATTERNS,

1
Full dress,
"white tie
and tails"

2
Dinner suit,
"black tie."
(Summer
version:
white jacket,
black formal
trousers)

3
Black suit

4
Navy
pinstripe

5
Navy
solid

12
Navy blazer,
smooth finish

13
Navy blazer,
"fuzzy" or
flannel
woolen

14
Sports jacket,
subtle wool
tweed. Camel
or gray
blazer.
Worn with tie.

15
Sports jacket,
heavier,
bolder
tweed. With
shirt and tie.
Worn with or
without
sweater.

16
Blazer or
tweed sports
jacket. Solid
or striped
shirt, worn
open, no tie.

NOTE: No suit pattern should be distinctly discernible from more than eight feet away. If it is obvious beyond that distance, it is too strident. Choose a subtler one.

● *White tie*. Unless you travel with the diplomatic set, there is little reason to own a full-dress suit. On those rare occasions when you are required to wear one, you'd do well to rent an outfit at the best rental agency in town.

● Dinner suit. Also called an evening suit or "black tie." (Currently it is not considered chic to call it a *tuxedo*. A waiter wears a tuxedo; his customer wears a dinner suit.) Styles and cuts change slowly from year to year, more noticeably over a six- or ten-year period, but then the pendulum swings back. Chapter 19 discusses black-tie dressing in full.

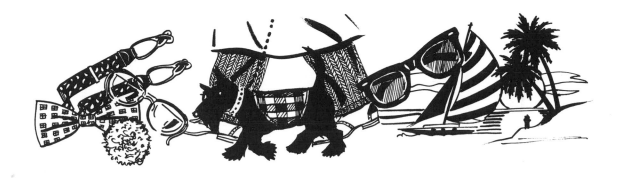

FORMAL TO CASUAL

6	7	8	9	10	11
Dark gray pinstripe	Dark gray solid	Medium to dark blue or gray. Small, subtle pattern; tick weave; smooth-finish self-weaves; mini-herring-bones.	Medium blue or medium gray; glen plaid	Medium to light blue or gray. (Not too light!)	Tan suit

17	18	19	20	21
Blazer or tweed sports jacket. Plaid shirt, no tie.	Blazer or tweed sports jacket. Knit polo shirt. Or "Miami Vice" look: sports jacket with T-shirt.	Casual clothes without sports jacket—with sweater or windbreaker	Casual clothes with jeans	Casual clothes with shorts

● **Patterns 4 through 11, and only those, are suitable for business wear.** A navy pinstripe, the most formal of business suits, is the uniform of CEOs of large corporations, bank presidents, and others who have reached the top. If worn daily, however, how can you top it for the really important days?

● *It is the shade of blue or gray,* rather than the pattern it may bear, that determines a suit's ranking on the formal-to-casual scale. Dark is equated with formality; medium tones are less dressy. This emphasizes the need to keep away from too-light blues and grays.

● *Blazers and sports jackets* have a hierarchy of their own, ranked chiefly by texture and the absence or subtlety of their patterns. Chapters 17 and 18 describe various components of casual and weekend wardrobes, and how to combine them.

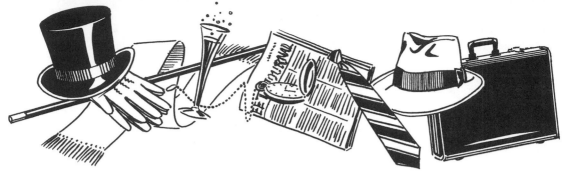

SHIRT PATTERNS,

1
"White tie" formal. Pleated front white evening dress shirt. Wing collar is traditional with white tie.

2
"Black tie" formal. Pleated front white (only) evening dress shirt—no ruffles. Point collar. Wing collars are worn, but are not as traditionally correct.

3
"White-on-white" or jacquard weave. Not generally appropriate for office wear. Some like this hyper-dressy look on weekends or vacations.

4
White shirt. Point collar, smooth broad-cloth fabric, worn with a collar pin.

5
White shirt. Point collar, smooth fabric, without collar pin.

12
Bengal stripes, navy and white or burgundy and white

13
Button-down striped oxford cloth

14
End-on-end weaves

15
Button-down broadly spaced stripes— pastels in summer, stronger colors in winter

16
Tattersalls or small checks

• Both white-tie and black-tie dressing dictate firmly the kind of tie you will wear with those shirts. Studs and cuff links, rather than buttons, are the way to go. Some fine European-influenced formal shirts come with a fly front and concealed buttons, eliminating any need for studs. No ruffles, please; they were questionable at any time, and have been totally taboo for several years.

• **In most industries, shirt patterns 4 through 11 are the only acceptable ones for business wear. In certain industries—notably communications, engineering, and entertainment—patterns 12 through 17 are also acceptable.**

• Patterns 8 and 9 are a toss-up for formality. They are about equal. Despite a nearly universal notion that a button-down oxford cloth shirt is correct with every suit and in every situation, it ranks eleventh on the shirt list. The disparity between the dressy number 4 pin striped suit and the number 11 button-down oxford cloth shirt is so wide that you really should reconsider wearing them together. The number 4 and 5 shirts are much better choices. If you like to wear button-down oxford shirts with everything, try one of the newer pinpoint oxford cloths or a button-down broadcloth.

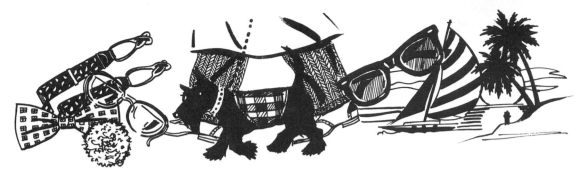

FORMAL TO CASUAL

6
Cream or light blue solid. Striped shirt with white background, fine blue or gray stripes, point collar.

7
White contrast collar, colored body (solid or striped), with or without collar pin

8
Button-down broadcloth, solids or stripes

9
Point collar pinpoint oxford cloth

10
Button-down pinpoint oxford cloth

11
Button-down oxford cloth, solid colors

17
Button-down chambrays and small checks

18
Plaid shirt worn with tie

19
Plaid shirt worn without tie

20
Knit polo shirt (with collar)

21
Knit T-shirt (without collar)

• *Broadcloth* is a smooth, plain, closely woven fabric. *Pinpoint oxford* is more tightly woven than conventional oxford cloth, yet has some of the same attractive texture. Smoother, luxurious, more expensive, it is a cross between broadcloth and oxford cloth. *Jacquard* is a type of weave that introduces a raised, sometimes intricate pattern into the cloth. Avoid it in white-on-white, colored tone-on-tone, and satin striped shirts for business wear. It is too slick a look. *Bengal stripes* are bold stripes, one sixteenth of an inch wide, often on broadcloth. Named for the similarly striped Bengal tiger, it is the boldest of all the classically accepted shirts. *End-on-end* is a pattern in which alternating white and colored yarns, usually blue, are woven both horizontally and vertically. This creates a tightly checkered, subtle suggestion of a pattern, yet a smooth texture. A classic staple in a complete wardrobe is *chambray,* in which white threads are woven across colored threads, giving a distinctive somewhat faded appearance to the fabric (something like a very lightweight denim). Chambray is nearly always blue, although other colors are occasionally seen. *Tattersall* is the name given to a weaving pattern in which dark-lined squares intersect with lighter-lined squares. The background is always light, most often white. It is a handsome, classic, slightly casual shirt, perfect for wear with a solid wool tie or open at the neck. Every wardrobe should include one blue end-on-end and one Tattersall shirt, for wear with everything from less formal suits to blazers or jeans.

1	2	3	4	5
White piqué bow tie	Black formal bow tie, smooth satin or grosgrain. (Occasionally a colored bow tie is substituted.)	Navy background, small white pindot in smooth silk	Hermès navy background, small white (or light blue) pattern in smooth silk	Navy foulard, small neat pattern in white, pearl gray, or light blue in smooth silk

11	12	13	14	15
Navy and white stripe in silk repp	Solid navy in smooth silk	Solid burgundy or crimson in smooth silk	Navy club in woven jacquard silk	Burgundy club in woven jacquard

21	22	23	24	25
Small neat pattern in silk and wool blends	Small pattern or paisley in wool challis (w)	Larger paisley in wool challis (w)	Solid in wool (w) or Viyella (w)	Stripes or solids cotton (s) or linen (s)

• **Patterns 3 through 25 are acceptable for business wear.** Ties marked (w) should be reserved for winter wear, and ones marked (s) worn only during the summer months.

• *Piqué* is a cotton fabric woven in a waffle or honeycomb pattern and used for white bow ties. It is worn only on the most formal of formal occasions with tails, in white-tie dressing.

• Avoid ties made of polyester; it is not an adequate substitute for silk, and does not make a good knot. It also pills from rubbing against your beard. Just as wool is the fabric for suits and cotton is the cloth for shirts, the best ties are made of silk.

• Tie fabrics with a heavy "hand"—a woolly, fuzzy touch—are best worn with heavier, winter-weight suitings and Harris tweed types of sports jackets.

• Higher on the formal scale are foulards (silk, or silk and cotton, with small, neat overall printed designs) and solid-color silks. When wearing correspondingly high-numbered suits and shirts, confine your tie choices to numbers 3 through 17 on the tie pattern chart.

• A club tie—a tie bearing small, embossed figures of a tennis racket or anchor or organizational insignia woven into a solid twill background—was originally the emblem of one's private club. It is acceptable and is generally worn with a blazer, but it does make a statement. The wearer is saying, "I went to Dartmouth" or "I own a sailboat." Accordingly, club ties, even if they represent an honest interest, have an air of affectation. My advice: Why bother? There are hundreds of other choices that are noncontroversial and equally attractive.

• A designer's logo or initials prominently embroidered on a tie are advertisements for that

FORMAL TO CASUAL

6
Other Hermès tie, any background color in smooth silk

7
Red foulard, small pattern in smooth silk

8
Yellow background foulard in smooth silk

9
Navy foulard, small red pattern in smooth silk

10
Navy foulard, small colored pattern in smooth silk

16
Other foulard colors in smooth silk

17
Navy, red, or burgundy stripe in smooth silk

18
Any of patterns 3–17 in browns

19
Solid silk shantung (s), "raw silk" (s), or ribbed silk

20
Small all-over paisley in smooth silk

26
Silk knit

27
Cotton madras (s), wool (w), or Viyella (w) plaid

28
Cotton (s) or wool (w) knit

designer. Why be a walking billboard? You neither gain status nor are paid rent for the use of your shirt front. In all, a poor deal and poor taste, in my view.

• A pattern's scale is important. The rule: The smaller the pattern, the more elegant the look. A small pindot is formal, a medium-sized dot is less so. A large, overscaled dot looks like part of a clown's costume. A small paisley is dressy and always proper; a large paisley is casual.

• You will find pages of information about ties—how they are made and how to select the right ones and get value for your dollars—in chapter 8. Here, a few definitions: *Repp* is a ribbed-silk fabric. The term is commonly used to describe a diagonally striped tie. *Regimental* stripes have a solid background color, with narrow bands of two or three colors alternating the length of the tie. *University* stripes are woven of a silk twill or ribbed fabric with equally wide bands of two colors. *Blazer* stripes have one dominant band, bisected by a brightly colored stripe, alternating with a narrower band of a third color. All are safe bets for business wear. *Paisley* is an overall, multi-colored design, Indian in origin and flavor, with a teardrop-shaped pattern. Small-design paisleys are fine for all business occasions. Larger patterns are at the extremely casual end of the acceptable range.

• Two wonderful tie fabrics that you can find only in the better shops are *ancient madder*, an all-silk tie fabric woven with a marvelously dusky cast to its colors, much like "film" on the freshest of Concord grapes, and a suedelike "hand"; and *silk crepe*, a light, soft, and luxurious fabric that has a smooth surface and is very dressy (a bit too formal for summer wear).

• Pronounce *challis* as *shal'-ee*. It is a smooth, lightweight wool or wool and cotton fabric, usually printed with an all-over pattern.

Corresponding charts immediately following the suit pages cover options for shirts and ties. **The numbering scheme of the first two charts is approximately the same,** so that a number 11 suit will coordinate neatly with a shirt in the 9–13 range. A tie in that middle range will be a good choice, too.

The numbers are not precise, they are approximate; but they are a reliable general guide. That is, numbers that are approximately the same on suit, shirt, and tie charts mean harmonious combinations. The numbers need not be identical, but a number 4 suit, number 17 shirt, and number 24 tie wouldn't work at all.

The Name of the Tie

A tie that is appropriate for business wear should have a name. It is usually a one-word name: foulard, paisley, dot, stripe, solid, or club. Even a plaid or a knit.

The one tie in a class by itself is a registered trademark. It is an Hermès tie from France. In a sense it can be described as a small, neat pattern printed on the finest silk fabric. But an Hermès tie is much more. These ties are recognized by other men who wear them, not because they bear any logo, but because of their distinctive and elegant patterns. Manufactured by the famed Parisian house of fine leather goods, suedes, and silks, they are probably the finest ties in the world. The average price is $60. "Outrageous!" you say. But think about it. What other item can you buy for $60 and know that you own the finest of its kind in the world?

The Diminishing Effect

You'll recall the warning note I sounded about the urge to merge among colors. A perfectly beautiful overall red pattern on a blue background is precisely the tie you want to be seen in, when you glance at it on your tie rack. But when seen from eight feet away, or from table 4 when you're on the speaker's platform, it is a nondescript, purplish color.

Pattern, too, can disappear or change in direct relationship to the viewer's distance. You might build your day's appearance on the rich, subtle complexity of a suit's blue or gray tick weave. (Those are minute, regular squares of soft blue or gray—no more than one sixty-fourth of an inch each—alternating with the dominant dark-color woolen fabric.) Because of the suit's character and pattern, you dress down otherwise: a point collar, pearl gray shirt, and a fine navy silk tie. You're perfect as you look in the mirror. But from across the room, to anyone with average vision, you look like a study in blue-gray monotony.

Watch carefully the diminishing effect inherent in other patterned suits as well—chalk stripes, glen plaids, even the lightest of pinstripes. And with shirts and ties, be aware that not only will *pattern* merge and meld at relatively short distances, but *texture* may very well disappear entirely. The ribbing in a silk repp or the weave of a club tie contributes to its sparkle across a lunch table or when seen in a television close-up. But across an auditorium floor it is gone, gone, gone.

Paradoxically you *want* your suit's pattern to become indistinct when seen from across the room. Any *suit* pattern that remains sharply visible at a distance of eight feet is too bold. "Horsey" is what it's called in the clothing trade.

The remedy for the diminishing effect lies in your choice of tie. If you are speaking to an audience of more than twenty people, wear a tie that has widely spaced, bold stripes. With a blue suit, your tie might have a navy background and wide yellow diagonal stripes bordered by a narrow white line, or a burgundy background dominated by medium blue stripes. From a distance, tie patterns such as these will still be visible.

How to Look at Color in a Pattern

I'm sure you have seen someone in a store examining a necktie so closely that it was only a few inches from his or her eyes, trying to determine the exact color in the smallest pattern or in one of the secondary stripes. That is not the way to decide if the colors match. Not that close examination isn't important; it's just that it doesn't work.

The way to view an item that you are trying to coordinate is to hold it at arm's length or, better yet, step back a bit. That is how others perceive it. The overall color effect of a pattern changes as you get farther away from it.

Try this experiment for yourself: Find a "goes with anything" tie in your closet—one that has a small, neat pattern of red, or red and white, on a blue background. Up close, the tie is a subtle blue and red foulard, appropriate for any business situation.

From a distance of a few feet, it still looks the same. Now stand in front of a mirror and move back a bit. The pattern disappears; the tie's color becomes purple to your eye. Step back even farther, and from across the room, the tie becomes brown.

This little exercise illustrates two principles. One, when you are selecting a tie in a store or at home, always hold it away from you. The second is: To check the color of a tie you plan to wear for a presentation to a group of people, stand back as far as you can from your mirror. Wear bold colors that are visible from a distance.

This principle is not confined to clothes. Several years ago I was at a friend's house on a day when a new carpet was being laid in an upstairs room. It was a rich blue with a yellow tweed pattern, custom-woven to the designer's exact specifications. The two colors were perfect matches for the blue and yellow furniture in the room.

My friend and I spent an hour talking together, then went upstairs anxious to see how terrific it all looked. I will never forget our shock at seeing that blue and yellow room with its luxurious new *green* carpet!

The designer, who should have known what you have already learned, was clearly responsible. My friend had to replace the carpet. Had the designer remembered to stand back a few feet to check the effect of her sample, she would have avoided a fiercely expensive mistake.

Put Your Color and Pattern Savvy
to the Test

The tips and principles for combining patterns and colors in this chapter are not ones that I made up. No, the combinations of clothing colors and patterns that send out messages of success, power, and importance are dictated by the upper levels of American businessmen. To prove that you are ready to play their game—*and win*—take the simple quiz that follows.* If you score well on it, you can be confident that you will score equally well in the real game you'll be dressing for on Monday morning.

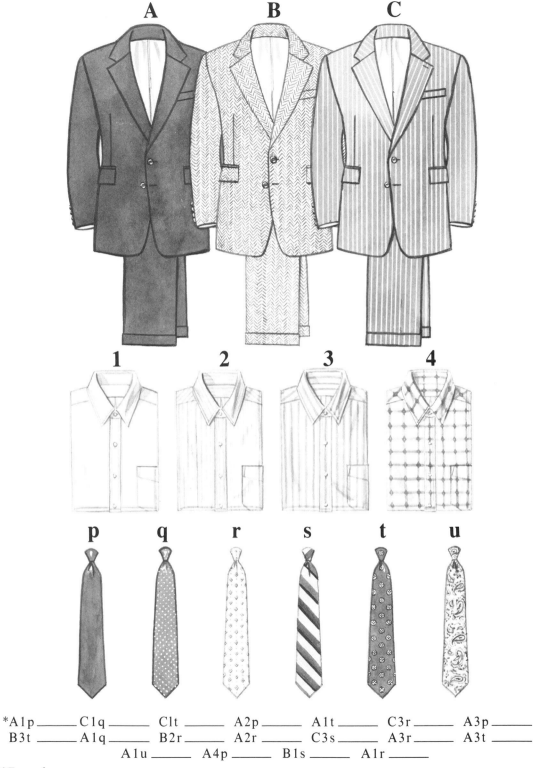

A	B	C
1	2	3	4
p	q	r	s	t	u

*A1p _____ C1q _____ C1t _____ A2p _____ A1t _____ C3r _____ A3p _____

B3t _____ A1q _____ B2r _____ A2r _____ C3s _____ A3r _____ A3t _____

A1u _____ A4p _____ B1s _____ A1r _____

*Example:
 Match suit (A) with shirt (1) and tie (p) and answer yes or no to the question: "Are you dressed for excellence?"

*Adapted from the *Donnelley Record,* issue 1979, no. 1, The Reuben H. Donnelley Corporation, and used with permission.

ANSWERS TO QUIZ

A 1 p

Yes, can be *very* sophisticated when color is used well.

B 3 t

No, too busy.

C 1 q

Yes, the "diplomat or chairman of the board look." Elegant. Too formal for some situations. Can be made less dressy by substituting a foulard (r) for the polka-dot (q) tie. A striped suit is limiting in terms of where you wear it and what you wear with it.

A 1 q

Yes, one of the most handsome, elegant looks, particularly when the polka dots are small and light-colored on a dark tie.

C 1 t

Yes, you'll knock 'em dead in this one.

B 2 r

No, never. Well, hardly ever. If the pattern of the suit is very subdued, such as a subtle herringbone or tweed, rather than a bold plaid or check, it *could* work. But it is generally best not to combine any three patterns. Since every rule has an exception, the exception to the never-wear-three-patterns-together rule is: A small, silk pocket square may introduce a third pattern. This is true because the item is so small, but it is not easy to do well.

A 2 p

Yes, the safest and surest combination. With reasonable care in selecting colors, you should *always* be able to do this well. Solid-color ties are most useful in navy, brown, and wine.

A 2 r

Yes and no. This is easy to do poorly, which is the way you usually see it. But annual reports are full of pictures of men in this combination. Harmonious color coordination is the important difference between unattractive and highly distinctive.

A 1 t

Yes, even Fred Astaire couldn't do it better.

C 3 s

No, you've got to be kidding!

C 3 r

No, no, no. Almost as bad as C 3 s.

A 3 r

No, this shirt requires a solid-color suit and tie or a spaced club tie (t).

A 3 p

Yes, a safe, smart way to be a bit bold and distinctive.

A 3 t

Yes, another way to be bold and distinctive, but more difficult to do than A 3 p.

A 1 u

Yes, the paisley tie is a great way to spark up a too-dull combination.

A 4 p

No, even though it is correct to combine one pattern with two plains, this type of shirt is *never* appropriate for business or professional wear—except for a formal luau.

B 1 s

Yes, particularly handsome when the shirt repeats the second, or less dominant, color in the suit. Example: With a subdued brown glen plaid suit with a blue line in the design, wear a blue shirt with a brown and blue tie. Brown and blue is a "successful"-looking color combination, particularly in dark brown and light blue or navy and camel. Avoid dark brown and dark blue.

A 1 r

Yes, a guarantee comes with this one. Though it is not particularly distinctive, it is always right. Almost every famous and successful man in the world has been photographed in this one.

11

Texture:
Your Secret Weapon

What Texture Says About You

Texture—the qualities of roughness or smoothness in fabrics—can present you to the world as trustworthy, safe, and reliable. Or they can peg you as slick and too smooth for comfort.

Even the words "He's too *smooth* and *slick—too glitzy*" are terms that describe textures. They have negative connotations. They do not say *serious, stable,* or *classic,* which is what your clothes should say about you. They definitely do not describe someone you would trust with your life savings.

Just take a look at Keith. In his own eyes, Keith presents a perfect appearance. In ours, it is too much. He is wearing a dark blue silk suit (smooth) and a white-on-white shirt (slick) and a shiny silk solid red or burgundy tie. His belt and shoes are made from the hide of the shiniest alligator that ever slithered up the Amazon. He wears a chunky, expensive gold watch on one wrist and a gold ID bracelet on the other. His hair is slicked back and smooth. Would you want him to date your sister or daughter?

How could we make Keith over, take away some of the glossy slickness and give him a softer finish? To start, we'd allow his hair to assume its natural texture and balance. His dark blue suit would be fine if we changed its texture to a wool, even to a smooth-textured wool. We'd get rid of that white-on-white shirt and substitute a white shirt in oxford cloth. The red or burgundy tie is fine, but I might prefer a matte finish rather than a shiny one.

Keith's alligator belt is perfectly acceptable. It has shine and elegance. But his alligator shoes are for social wear at best; I'd think long and hard before making such a large investment in a questionable item.

Although I find a slim gold watch to be one of the nicest touches a man can wear, the big gold watch isn't wrong. What is wrong is the predictability of it. (You think I am exaggerating? One summer I lectured on a cruise ship sailing around the Mediterranean. The men on the cruise were Americans, winners of an incentive program for selling tons of industrial equipment. I have never seen such a concentration of large gold watches in my life. And the number of watches encircled with diamonds was dazzling.)

Keith's original look, an unrelieved collection of too-smooth textures, said, "Cold. Elusive. A hard guy to trust." After our changes, he could come across as warm, responsive, and trustworthy.

In realistic terms, texture *does* make a statement. Smooth textures have an air of hardness, crispness, and power. They can give you a cool, somewhat standoffish quality.

Soft textures—woolens, open weaves, nubby finishes—seem warmer and more friendly.

A Balancing Act

The secret of using textures advantageously is *balance:* balance between contrast and repetition, and between rough and smooth.

Too much contrast can be jarring. Too much repetition can be boring. Not all of your looks need stay in one mode. Everyone should exhibit some variety while keeping a balance. There are times to make it clear you are in control—and other times when you would do well to appear to be a facilitator, a "let's work together" kind of person.

In the clothes power game, *smooth textures parallel dark (control) colors; rough textures parallel lighter (facilitator) colors.*

A smooth broadcloth shirt goes with a silk tie and logically is worn with an elegant, smooth-finished dressy suit. At the opposite end of the texture scale, a woven oxford cloth shirt goes with a wool tie and a lamb's wool sweater; they coordinate perfectly with a rough Harris tweed sports jacket and a pair of flannel trousers.

Smooth with smooth, and rough with rough. That's a way to start. Now let's say you have a reason for wanting to vary that rule.

Your company is having a meeting at a conference center in the suburbs. Or the boss is having an autumn party outdoors. You plan to wear a tweed sportscoat. You could wear the expected chambray shirt

---

Three Easy Rules About Texture

You already know **Rule 1,** but it won't hurt to repeat it. **Wear rough textures with rough textures; wear smooth with smooth.**

Rule 2: The smoother the texture, the dressier the look. Think about suits. A fine dark blue wool and silk, perhaps double-breasted, might be seen on a State Department senior officer, one attending an international conference. Woolens and worsteds, somewhat less smooth, are dressy enough for most business occasions. And flannels or muted tweeds, considerably rougher than silk, are about the least formal suit fabrics admissible for ordinary business wear.

Although Rule 1 calls for rough with rough and smooth with smooth, **some contrast is essential.** That's **Rule 3.** A deft touch, a subtle one, is required for balance. Usually it can be achieved through your choice of shirt and necktie pattern. Steer between the hazards of a boring, dull look or, even worse, a too-slick one.

and knit tie, but it would be a touch too informal for the occasion. The jacket is appropriate, but your instincts tell you the shirt and the tie are not quite right for the occasion. *You can adjust the texture to define how dressy you want to look.* You decide on a button-down pinpoint oxford cloth shirt (number 10 on the chart on page 139) that is a shade dressier than a standard oxford cloth (11) and several steps dressier than the chambray (17). Then choose a tie in a wool paisley (22), rather than the less formal wool knit (28).

You have taken control. You have adapted the rule and made it work for you.

Texture Combinations That Win at Work

Perfect combinations are neither too smooth and formal for a work atmosphere nor too rough and informal for the office. They combine a bit of the best of both.

- Suits of finely woven worsted are worn with cotton shirts—your choice of smooth broadcloth, slightly less smooth pinpoint oxford cloth, more textured oxford cloth, or end-on-end weaves. These work with any variety of silk neckties.
- Suits of woolen flannel are fuzzier in texture than worsteds and consequently less formal.
- Wool ties, both woven and knit, are too rough in texture and mood for a smooth-finished suit, especially one that is dark gray or blue. Here color and texture reinforce each other. If both are formal, as in smooth textures and dark colors, the overall effect becomes even more formal.
- Just as color reinforces texture, so does pattern. A striped or tattersall shirt—both less formal than one that is white or a solid color—would work well with the casual texture of a flannel suit. That is why certain shirts—notably bold plaids, broad stripes, and darker colors—are considered to be "blazer shirts." They work wonderfully with the sophisticated informality of a blazer. Generally they are not appropriate with business suits.

To help train your eye, try this experiment: Select two shirts of contrasting textures from your closet. One shirt might be a smooth cotton broadcloth, the other a rougher button-down oxford cloth. Now choose several different ties: your dressiest silks, a striped repp, perhaps a wool solid, and a knit tie. Place each tie against the shirts. Your eyes will tell you which ones are too dressy for the oxford cloth and which go better with the elegance of the fine broadcloth. What a difference texture makes!

Spirit

Sophisticated mixing and matching involves combining items compatible in pattern, texture, and "spirit." The concept of *spirit* is simple: It might be defined as "mood." It has to do with suitability. You wouldn't wear brown topsiders with a pinstripe suit, would you?

But you might wear any of these three typical groupings. The patterns, textures, and *spirit* all go together perfectly. *First,* for that perennial Dartmouth look, a casual outfit might include a sports jacket, a blue

---

Textures, Colors, Patterns—and Pigeonholes

The texture of your clothes is in many ways a reflection of your personality. Some personalities just naturally suggest certain moods or certain clothes, and dressing in any other way seems incongruous.

You may be the formal or dressy type. But more than likely, you think of yourself as relaxed. Even so, in your approach to business and your climb upward, it is unlikely that you want to be pigeonholed as casual and "tweedy" (unless you're in academia, where tweediness may be exactly the image you want). In business circles why leave the category of the "in-charge type" to others?

It makes a great deal of sense to decide what you want, and to orchestrate carefully the look that you wish to project. *Textures,* along with *colors* and *patterns,* are instruments to make it all work for you.

oxford cloth shirt, a Shetland sweater, a wool tie, loafers, and argyle socks. *Second,* a much more formal, authoritative grouping could include a dark pinstripe suit, a white broadcloth shirt, a silk tie, fine cotton lisle hose, and wing-tip shoes. This is the boardroom look. *Finally,* the spirit of the most formal group, the black-tie look, is elegance. You might wear a black evening suit with satin lapels, a pleated shirt, a silk bow tie, silk hose, and black patent-leather pumps.

Are You Visible Among Business Leaders?

To some degree, when you dress for business you are wearing a uniform. You are wearing the kind of suit that successful executives wear, and that they expect to see others wearing. In style and cut and essential details, your shirt will be the prescribed shirt. And your tie, theoretically one of many patterns and colors available to you, is exactly the kind of tie that leaders want to see. They know it is right, because they themselves wear ties practically identical to it.

So, a cynic might observe, why not go whole hog? Why not wear a uniform? If you did, I'll tell you what would happen. The true leaders, the powerful men at the apex of success, would *still* stand out, thanks to the perfect tailoring of their jackets, their authoritative manners, their grooming and carriage.

Businessmen don't have to wear uniforms. Like the eagles and stars on an officer's shoulders, one man's clothing says to another's, "I'm important." And since you now know as much as the next man—probably considerably more—about combining colors, patterns, and textures, you will emerge as one of those from whom the power flows.

12

The Coats
That Create a
Great First Impression

Below is a list of eight styles of coats that you might consider as important components of your wardrobe. But you can survive—even flourish—with only one. In that case, try to make it the one I have listed first.

• **A raincoat with a removable lining.** Don't think about a dark-colored one such as navy or black, one that "doesn't show soil marks too quickly." Confine your selection to khaki or tan. And start the selection process in an absolutely topflight store, one that carries the Burberry line of coats.

You may not decide to buy this Rolls-Royce of coats. But once you try one on, you will know what the best looks and feels like, and have a reference point for judging other brands and models. An all-cotton, top-of-the-line Burberry trench coat—complete with its recognizable wool collar, epaulets, belt, an impressive brass loop or two, and a button-in wool liner—will cost slightly less than $600. A blend of cotton and polyester with similar styling is priced at about $425. Other models move comfortably downward in cost: A single-breasted version with the distinctive Burberry plaid lining is about $350, and an extremely lightweight travel raincoat is priced at the low end of the scale, $250.

For added dash in a trench coat, today's style suggests that you knot the belt, rather then slip it through the buckle. If you are short or somewhat heavy, a double-breasted coat may accentuate width at the expense of height. For that reason, you may do better choosing a single-breasted coat, which will elongate your figure.

Burberrys are seldom on sale. The styles do not change, so the retailer has no need to mark down this season's unsold merchandise. He packs the coats away in the stockroom until next year and perhaps even raises the price a little to keep pace with inflation. It is exactly this never-out-of-style quality that makes the coat a good investment. Burberrys last for about eight years of normal wear. (Incidentally, the Burberry you buy in London is far less expensive than one bought here, and it is still made in the original Burberry workrooms. Your savings can help justify the trip.)

Sharing the top honors in raincoats with Burberry, according to many well-dressed European men, is the 100 percent cotton model made by Aquascutum of London. If you are like many men, you rely on your raincoat to take you through travel situations and the many climate changes travel can bring. One veteran traveler (on the high seas, at least) I talked to was Captain Gregory C. Avdelas, Master of the s.s. *Royal Odyssey* of the Royal Cruise Line. He is a great admirer of the Aquascutum raincoat, or gabardines, as they are called in Europe: "I can wear it sitting on a plane for three hours and never look wrinkled."

· **A wool topcoat.** If you already have a good raincoat and need a second cold-weather coat, a wool or wool and cashmere blend topcoat is your next choice. Slightly on the formal side, it should be dark blue or dark gray, either a solid color or a muted herringbone tweed. Select single- or double-breasted styling, depending on your preference. (Re-

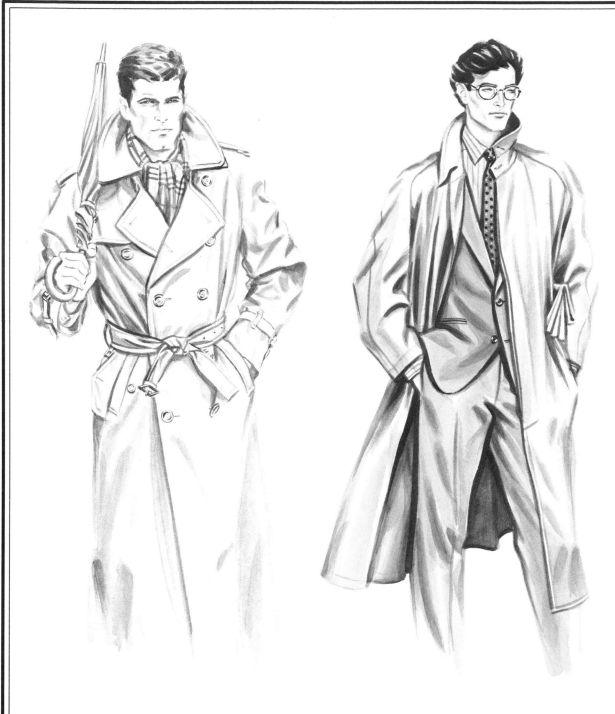

Double-breasted trench coat   Single-breasted raincoat

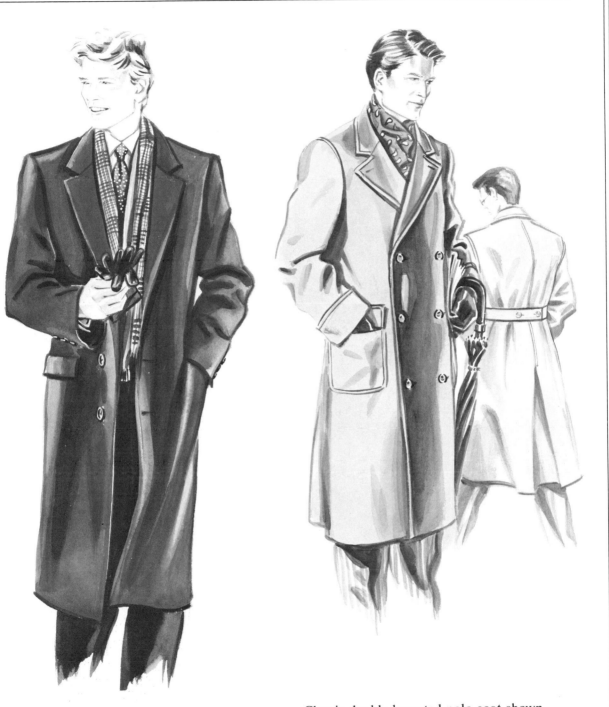

Wool topcoat

Classic double-breasted polo coat shown
with belted back

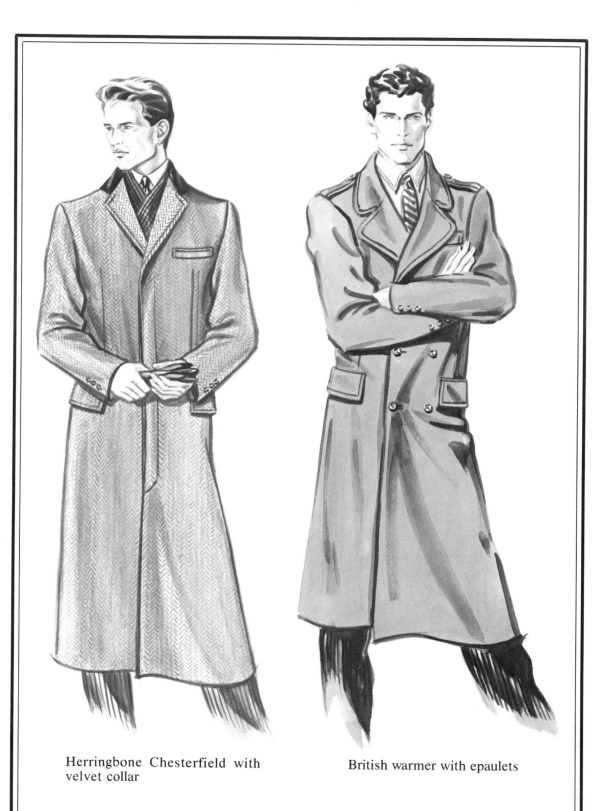

Herringbone Chesterfield with
velvet collar

British warmer with epaulets

serve the possibility of a second light-colored coat—a camel hair—for further down your list.)

Unless you live in Duluth or a similarly subarctic climate, today's business demands do not require a heavier coat, known as an overcoat. You are in and out of cars and buildings, and there are few hours in an average year when you will need the stifling warmth of an old-fashioned overcoat.

No coat should be purchased without a full try-on. Wear a suit jacket under the coat. Assure yourself of free movement and uncramped fit. Also look at the length: Coats should extend well below the knee. Do not be influenced by a salesman who tells you that this season's style calls for anything shorter. It doesn't. In fact, in recent years men's coats are being worn longer than they were several years ago. If the coat has a back vent, it should hang straight and closed when the coat is buttoned.

· **A polo coat (camel-hair topcoat).** It might be genuine camel, or it might be a camel-colored cashmere and wool blend, or all wool. Pure cashmere is wonderfully warm and luxurious, but too perishable for most everyday uses. Your tan wool coat is usually double-breasted, loosely belted in the back.

· **A Chesterfield topcoat.** These dressy, warm, British-styled coats are distinguished by a fitted cut, slightly suppressed at the waist, and a collar that is customarily velvet. I recommend dark gray, or a small gray herringbone pattern, as a strong first choice. Second choice is navy. When tailored of solid black wool, Chesterfields create a marvelously dressy image, but are a touch too formal for everyday business wear. In some circles they could be considered an affectation.

· **A wool tweed coat.** These rather casual coats are easy to wear over suits, blazers, and sports clothes. They are made in lighter colors and bolder tweeds than wool topcoats and are tremendously durable.

· **A British warmer.** This military-style coat extends only to the knees. Slightly shorter and made of melton (a thickly woven, virtually windproof type of woolen fabric), it is more casual than the other coats listed above. It is usually seen in navy, taupe, or khaki, and can substitute for a stadium coat. Epaulets contribute to the sporty look.

· **A very light raincoat for travel wear.**

· **A wool or cashmere coat with a fur collar.** Last on the list and certainly not for everyone is a dark wool coat with a beaver, nutria, or raccoon collar. This coat is uncontested for dressing beyond the crowd. If your closet and your budget can accommodate one, do not ruin the effect by buying a light-colored or twill-like texture for your fur-collared coat. Solid dark blue or charcoal gray is the ideal choice. As for the collar, utilitarian furs are the rule for men's coats.

13

Accessories That Provide the Winning Edge

Granted that your suit, shirt, and tie constitute 90 percent of your business clothing's total effect. But, oh, the importance of that other 10 percent! Your shoes, scarf—even your wallet—and perhaps a dozen other items complete the picture of excellence that you project. They are a tip-off to your success. We'll examine them one by one.

Shoes

What are the key indicators that a man really knows how to dress with style and taste? My answer has always been, "His shoes, his watch, and his tie." Although shoes may not seem to have as immediate an impact as a "power watch," they are important. Consider two men wearing the same $400 suit. One wears an inexpensive pair of black demi-boots; the other wears Brooks Brothers black cap-toe oxfords. They project two vastly different impressions.

Shoes, like neckties, should be the best you can afford. The difference shows, and you can feel it, too. Expensive shoes are usually comfortable shoes.

From Wing-Tips to Loafers, a Rolex to a Timex

Think of the thousands of types, varieties, and brands of men's apparel and specialty items available to you in any men's-wear store. They are all yours to choose from.

When making your choice, you'd do well to keep in mind Stanley Marcus's precepts on *simplicity.* In his book *Quest for the Best,* Marcus observes, "Simplicity in clothes serves as a foil . . . oversimplicity results in blandness; overdecoration is chaos."

Add to that the caution that a too-meticulous match is equally a mistake. Shoes and belts, suspenders and ties should *coordinate,* but not match exactly. Be alert to too studied or contrived an appearance.

Two kinds of shoes are acceptable for the world of business: *lace-up* and *slip-on.* Both are crafted here or abroad of smooth, supple leathers, and both are best when they are simple, straightforward, and free of unnecessary decorative touches. The colors that men in positions of authority wear are black, dark brown, and mahogany (or cordovan). Only those colors are proper for business footwear. Navy, gray, and tan are unacceptable.

• **Lace-up shoes.** In general, lace-up shoes are known as *oxfords.* Dressier ones have slightly thinner soles and heels, supple, shiny leather uppers, and four pairs of eyelets for the laces. Heavy, waterproof shoes suitable for a walk through the English countryside are not regarded as necessary for a day spent in a carpeted, air-conditioned office.

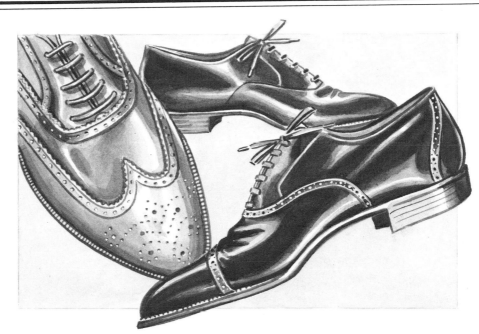

Lace-up shoes *(clockwise, beginning left):* classic wing tip; plain lace-up; cap-toed lace-up

Wing-tip oxfords are classic. The hallmark perforations on their caps and sides are made by various manufacturers in distinctive patterns, one differing ever so slightly from the other. Black wing tips are exactly right for pinstripe suits and any dressy dark blue or gray suit.

The *cap-toe oxford* has a thick, rounded welt across its toe. It, too, is appropriate with business suits that tend toward formality. Wing tips and cap-toes are the only two styles of shoes on which perforations are appropriate.

The *plain-toe oxford* is an anomaly. In cordovan or rich dark brown it is perfect with brown tweeds or a tan summer suit. Yet in black it is even more dressy than either of the other oxford styles—and in a pinch can double as black-tie footwear. True evening shoes are correctly made of thin, highly glossed, black patent leather. Today they need not always be patent leather; some of the better stores now sell formal pumps made of soft black calf. But patent-leather shoes of any kind are worn only as part of formal wear.

Suede shoes, when worn by a man who is knowledgeable of the nuances of dress—particularly one who enjoys a 1930s or British influence—elicit the phrase "Oh, of course! He buys his clothes in London."

Suede oxfords are found in some of the finest shoe shops, but they are understood and accepted in only very limited circles. My advice is to steer clear of them for business wear unless you see the top men in your establishment wearing them. Even then, proceed with caution.

· **Slip-on shoes.** Only in the mossiest of traditionalist circles are slip-on shoes considered less appropriate for business wear than lace-ups, and even in those enclaves, the slip-on is making inroads. The basic slip-on is a *classic loafer,* a version of what used to be called a penny loafer, but worn, of course, without pennies. One or more pairs of dark brown, mahogany, or black, gleamingly polished, are standbys that should be in every wardrobe. They go with all but the dressiest blue suits.

Tassel loafers substitute two small tassels of leather for the penny band of classic loafers. They should not have any perforations. In black they project a dressy image, but they are insufficiently formal for ultra-dressy occasions. They are totally out of place when worn with formal clothes.

Similar to tassel loafers, but with a fringed tongue of leather instead of the tassels, are *kilt (or shawl) loafers.* If you intend to own more than two pairs of loafers, you might consider the variety that this classic style imparts to a wardrobe.

Gucci has become a generic name for stylish loafers with a thin band of brass over the instep. In the original and in most copies, it is a piece of harness brass—actually a horse bit—that gives a distinctive air to these shoes. Gucci-styled loafers are another alternative to the slip-on shoe, but because of the brass decoration they are not appropriate for formal business or evening wear.

Permutations of the loafer abound. They have an eye-catching buckle here, an extra bit of brass there; sometimes a textured surface. Avoid them. Simplicity is the key to good taste in all things, and nowhere more so than in shoes. Running counter to desirable understatement are white shoes of any kind, worn at any time in the business world. Boots are almost as undesirable. An exception is made for western boots—cowboy boots worn by westerners—but only if the boots are made of the finest leather and are free of ornamentation.

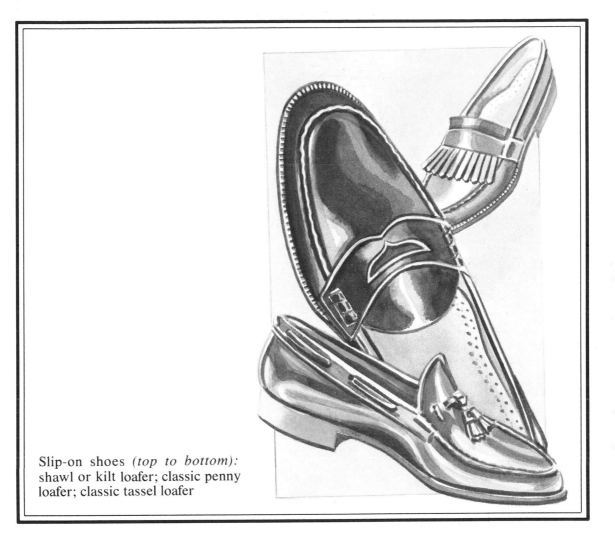

Slip-on shoes *(top to bottom):* shawl or kilt loafer; classic penny loafer; classic tassel loafer

Your shoe collection. When you locate a pair of shoes made of top-quality leather and with faultless workmanship and design, don't be surprised at the price tag. Paying upwards of $100 for a pair of shoes is not exorbitant in today's marketplace. I would suggest that you invest in three pairs as your core shoe wardrobe:

1 pair black oxfords
1 pair black simple slip-ons
1 pair dark brown or cordovan oxfords or slip-ons, in which you feel especially comfortable

Having invested a considerable amount in shoes, go the extra step and buy a set of shoe trees for each pair. After shoes have been dampened by rain or snow, they crinkle and tend to crack when drying if they are not set out to stretch properly on shoe trees. Frequent polishing is another

---

We've all made mistakes by hiring the wrong people. In an interview, I look beyond the résumé. For me, shoes are a dead giveaway for certain personality traits. By that I mean:

- You can tell a person's economic status; you can tell if the shoes are expensive or not.
- You can tell if a person is meticulous or not by observing whether the shoes are well cared for, polished, or in need of new heels. If they are shabby, then the person is obviously not one who is attuned to details. He's often the same person who overlooks important details in business.
- You can tell by the styling of the shoe whether or not the person is a trendy type. For example, if he wears a brogue, then he's probably a serious businessman. A less conservative shoe might indicate a more creative, artistic type—the type you'd get ideas from.
- Color is another strong indication of how a person feels about himself. A black shoe is a more sober indication with a gray suit. However, a person who knowingly wears a brown shoe with a gray flannel suit can show that he really knows how to dress. It's a wonderful look that displays he has a good sense of color and knows how to use it with sophistication.

The whole thing wrapped together is an indication of how the person sees himself. Shoes are a very strong statement of personality.

> —ROGER BAUGH, men's clothing
> designer, twice named to the
> International Best-Dressed List,
> 1983–84, 1985–86

essential. Those two easy chores will guarantee years of top-rate condition for any shoe that was constructed properly in the first place.

Allowing shoes to "rest" a few days between wearings also increases their life. This is another reason for expanding your shoe wardrobe to the extent your budget allows.

Socks

Business custom has removed almost all but two elements from your sock-buying decisions: Socks should be over the calf; their color should be solid and dark. There must never be any skin showing when you sit down and cross your legs. It is true that many men do wear short socks, just as many men wear short-sleeved business shirts. But a well-dressed man wears his socks to the calf or over it.

With blue or gray suits, black socks are worn. Navy blue can be substituted for black, though the shade should be so dark that you are probably the only one who will know it. Dark brown socks are worn only with brown shoes; never with black shoes.

Europeans and some adventuresome Americans sometimes move away from the solid, dark-color rule in socks. I have admired subtle tweeds, bird's-eye, and mini-herringbone patterns in their hose, in dark gray and burgundy as well as in blue and brown. These understated patterns are not easy to find, but they can be worth the effort. Bolder patterns such as argyle, and socks in lighter colors are best left for casual wear.

The sock fabrics preferred by most businessmen are lightweight wool, fine cotton lisle, and nylon. The lighter the weight and the smoother the weave, the dressier the sock. Blends of wool and nylon dry quickly and give long wear. Cashmere socks are warm and delicately luxurious, but they tend to develop holes quickly. When combined with nylon to reinforce the toes and heels, however, cashmeres are luxurious and practical.

A word about garters: If you confine yourself to over-the-calf lengths in your socks, you won't need them. But if you select calf-length socks for business wear and they tend to droop, garters will save the day.

Matching Suits, Shoes, and Socks		
Suit	Basic, Guaranteed Safe Shoe/Sock Choice	Interesting Variations
Gray suit	Black shoes, black socks	Dark brown shoes, charcoal gray or dark brown socks Cordovan shoes, dark gray socks
Navy suit	Black shoes, black or navy socks	Cordovan shoes, navy socks
Tan suit	Dark brown shoes, dark brown socks	Cordovan shoes, tweedy brown or burgundy socks Medium rich brown shoes, dark brown socks
Navy blazer, gray trousers	Black shoes, black, navy, or charcoal gray socks	Cordovan shoes, navy or dark gray socks
Navy blazer, camel or khaki trousers	Cordovan shoes, dark brown socks	Cordovan shoes, navy socks

Belts

With belts, less is more. A fine strip of supple, well-finished leather and a plain, understated metal buckle are all that a belt should be. Whether black or brown, a belt should be in the same color family as your shoes, although they need not match them exactly.

Men often discover that the belt they have purchased is too small. Since manufacturers size belts rather strangely, you must move up one size from your actual waist size when buying a belt. (The same is true for underpants.) Thus, if your waist measures 32 or 33, your belt size should be 34. Always try on a belt in the store and choose one that fits you comfortably when buckled through the middle hole.

Opting for a showy or decorative belt buckle is not wise. The V-shaped cut of suit lapels and a carefully combined shirt and tie selection are calculated to draw people's attention to your face. There is no logical reason to draw their attention to your waistline. Eschew turquoise and silver buckles. Keep away from buckles with designers' initials. Stay with quiet, tasteful belts that hold up your trousers and have no messages to send.

Suspenders

Suspenders, or braces, add dash to an outfit. With today's emphasis on pleated trousers, suspenders are seeing a rebirth of popularity.

Suspenders help trousers hang better. When you wear them, your trousers should be ever so slightly larger at the waist; in that way, they are suspended from the shoulders. This size adjustment can be made at the same time that your tailor sews in the six buttons necessary for wearing your new suspenders. Never wear clip-on suspenders. All of the sophistication is lost if you wear those metal clips—the kind created to attach children's mittens to their snowsuits.

As the oft-heard expression tells us, wearing a belt *and* suspenders offers the ultimate in safety. However, I don't advise it. Wear one or the other, but both at the same time is overkill. To make a bit of a fashion statement, the color and pattern of your suspenders should coordinate with both your shirt and your necktie. Three pairs—solid or dominantly dark blue, dark red, and gray—would give you all the coordinating colors you need. (You shouldn't feel that three pairs are your limit, however. One of my clients dominates a specialized area of finance. Wearing a different pair of suspenders every day has become his trademark. I have spent as many as four or five hours coordinating these items with shirts and ties, avoiding a too-perfect match but still giving him the variety he enjoys.)

Hats

The felt hat has never gone completely out of style, but its adherents have been a slim lot: primarily older men whose ideas of proper dress have not wavered over the decades. Since the Kennedy days, young men have preferred to go bareheaded. Today, happily, hats seem to be back in style. They have become a way of making a personal statement, and are seen more often on dapper dressers than on conservative ones.

If you should decide on a felt hat, look at the darker shades of gray before making your choice. Go to one of the older, better stores in town; it probably carries this year's line of classic fedoras (the felt hat's official name) bearing the Stetson label. Let the salesman show you a perfect fit and the perfect angle at which to wear it, in a style that flatters the lines of your face.

Tweed caps are another way to keep warm, but they are more appropriate for casual than for business wear. If you do wear a cap, it ought to be genuine British tweed, have a moderate-sized bill, and fall into the darker end of the blue-gray spectrum. Not as attractive or as acceptable, but indisputably warm, are fur hats. If you do choose to wear fur, it should be real and not a *faux* fur.

Gloves

Lucky the man who receives a pair of fine leather gloves for Christmas or his birthday! Luckier still he who receives two pairs. Good gloves, in pigskin or calfskin or any soft, durable leather, unlined or lined in cashmere, bear price tags of $40 and up. Your best gloves should be reserved for dress wear only, as any stressful use will scuff and scar the fine leather.

Thin gloves are a better choice than thick ones, as they won't stretch your coat pockets when stored there. Dull, rather than shiny, finishes are preferred. Wear dark brown gloves with camel coats and tweeds and black gloves with blue or gray suits and coats. Gray suede gloves are reserved for evening wear.

Scarves

The current popularity of scarves is surprisingly logical. A scarf keeps you warm, adds a touch of style and flair, and keeps the inside collar of your topcoat clean. Some of today's fashion-forward double-breasted coat styles are cut so low in front that a scarf is almost essential to prevent the suit lapels from showing.

Your choice of fabrics and colors is almost unlimited, as you can either repeat the color of your coat—but don't match the shade exactly— or wear a handsome contrast. Fine, soft woolens with a flannel-like surface are favorites; so are wool knits with a more textured surface. With a gray coat, a solid gray in a lighter shade would be smart, as would a solid burgundy. Or with the same coat, you might choose a plaid: gray and blue, gray and off-white, or gray and burgundy.

A white wool or cashmere scarf can dress up a dark coat for evening wear. The most elegant of all scarves is dark cashmere on one side, with a silk pattern, usually paisley or a foulard, on the other. An expensive investment, it should last forever. The most formal of all scarves is just that: a formal white silk scarf, worn exclusively as a dapper touch with black-tie evening wear.

Pocket Squares and Handkerchiefs

Pocket squares are silk in solid colors or all-over patterns—usually paisley or a small foulard. Handkerchiefs are white linen, freshly laundered and always ironed. Some men who would never wear a silk pocket square are comfortable with a linen handkerchief in their breast pocket. Other more conservative dressers will wear neither. Alan Flusser, the men's clothing designer, once told me, "The pocket was put there for a purpose—and it was not to collect debris."

Your aim with a colored square is to complement both the color and pattern of your necktie, but not to match the pattern exactly.

How do you coordinate, but not match? Here's an example: Consider a blue suit, a white or light blue shirt, and a red tie that has a small blue dot or blue foulard pattern. A good choice for a silk pocket square would be a navy background with a large-scaled red paisley pattern. Another possibility: a tan suit, blue shirt, blue-and-brown-striped tie with a pocket square in a dark brown and light blue all-over small foulard or pindot pattern.

With a pocket square you can experiment with introducing a third pattern into your outfit. If you are wearing a subtly striped suit *or* shirt, you can wear a patterned tie and pocket square. The amount of third

HOW TO WEAR POCKET SQUARES AND HANDKERCHIEFS

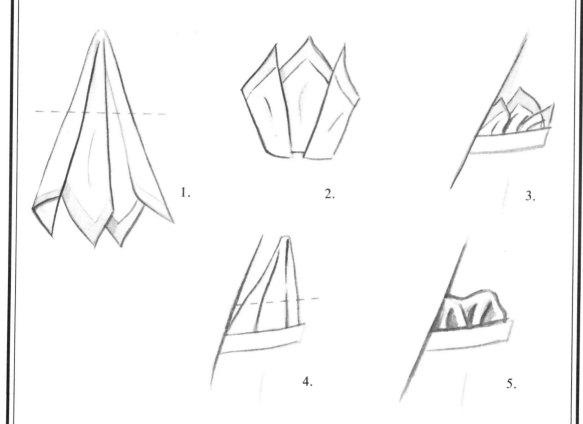

1. 2. 3.

4. 5.

Wearing a silk pocket square or a linen or cotton handkerchief in the breast pocket can add a dash of color or a bit of polish to an outfit. It is important to remember not to arrange it too precisely; a jaunty, slightly casual air is the effect you are trying to achieve. There are two ways of wearing this look:

1. First, open the square and put your index finger in the center. With your other hand, grasp the square at this center point and allow the four corners to fall naturally.
2. Fold this in half.
3. Poke square into pocket with the folded part down so that the points are up and showing slightly, not too much. Do *not* work too much at arranging these points. (It should not look like a picket fence.)
4. *Or,* after step 1, place square into pocket with the points facing down, fold in half at dotted line.
5. Poke single point into pocket, allowing the soft, slightly puffed center part of the square to show. This is a useful way to wear a patterned square when the border is too plain or you particularly want the center colors to show.

pattern seen in a pocket square is so slight and can be so well coordinated that the avoid-three-patterns rule can bend sufficiently to admit it.

Pictured opposite are the two ways to wear a pocket square. After folding it loosely to achieve four points, tuck it in your pocket—points up or points down. Either way, let it peek out of your pocket only a slight bit, and don't arrange it too precisely. Casual is the right tone.

Jewelry

The only pieces of jewelry appropriate for business dress are your watch, cuff links, wedding or signet rings, and your collar pin. In all cases, *simplicity* is the watchword.

• **Watches.** If you like sporty watches—the kind with stopwatch and calculator and other features—you need two watches: one for fun and one to wear to work. The best watch for business wear is the finest, most simply styled gold or stainless-steel watch that you can afford. A good leather strap is the classic choice, but gold- or silver-toned bands are chosen by many upper-level businessmen. Avoid inexpensive types of metal expansion bands. Dial faces are preferable to digital displays, and the face should be clean and unadorned, with no gems or decorations marring the neat lines of the timepiece.

• **Rings.** Here is where I urge caution. Of course, a wedding ring is always right. A signet ring is generally acceptable, especially if it is a family heirloom (or a tradition you have chosen to inaugurate). But a school ring may be out of place in your firm. See what top executives in your firm wear and be guided by their example.

• **Cuff links.** French cuffs are sometimes considered a bit showy, especially by men employed in conservative industries. At the very least, they consider French cuffs an annoyance, and they tell me that the links are just one more thing that they don't want to be bothered with in the morning.

French cuffs are dressier than barrel cuffs, and perhaps too dressy for some outfits. You might like to wear barrel cuffs for work and reserve your French-cuffed shirts for more social occasions.

If you have opted to wear barrel cuffs, fine; just do not wear those fake covers that clip over cuff buttons and masquerade as cuff links. They are phony and easily detected.

. . . As Big As the Ritz

Did you know that not for any price will Tiffany & Co. make a diamond ring for a man?

Their tradition insists that a gentleman does not wear a diamond ring.

A few years ago I was lecturing at a banker's convention in Palm Springs. At a large dinner one evening, I was seated at a table with seven other people, all bankers and their wives. Everyone was introduced; however, as often happens, I missed a few of the names. One of the men was well built, wearing traditional bankers' garb (navy suit, white shirt, and striped tie), but something was totally incongruous: He was wearing a mammoth diamond ring. Even more odd: As the evening progressed, men kept coming over to our table and asking for his autograph. I listened more carefully. He was Rocky Bleier of football fame, and the ring was his third Super Bowl ring. I decided that in that case it was just fine!

If you wear French cuffs, any simple, tasteful style of link will do, provided it is not too big or flashy and has no clear stones. If your watchband is silver, stay with silver-toned cuff links. With a gold watchband, wear gold cuff links. The finest cuff links are the "Edwardian" type, which actually link two identical pieces, rather than the customary single piece of jewelry attached to a clip-on device. Another option is paired silk knots, priced at about $5 in fine men's stores. They are in favor today as a substitute for conventional sets of links.

• **Collar pins.** If your shirts are designed for wearing with a pin through two eyelets in the collar, you have a choice of *straight bar* or *safety pin* types. The straight bar is somewhat dressier, having either round or cube screw-on ends. Wear it in gold or silver, depending on the shade of your watchband and cuff links.

You might substitute a *collar bar* for the eyelet fastener if you are wearing a straight point collar (one with no small embroidered holes in it). The bar is simply slid onto the collar, pulling it down and giving the shirt a trim and rather dapper look. Collar bars are never worn with button-down or spread (Windsor) collars. Collar pins and bars are among the most effective and least expensive touches a man can add to enhance his overall look.

· **Tie pins, tie tacks, and stick pins** are currently out of fashion—foolishly so, in my opinion, because it does not make sense for your tie to flap in the breeze or swing into your soup. This vogue of not wearing a tiepin is sure to leave us in a few years. For now, don't wear a tiepin, but don't discard any attractive ones that may be in your drawer.

To anchor your tie without the aid of a tiepin, slip the narrow end through the small loop of fabric sewn on the wide end. In most cases, it is the manufacturer's label; sometimes, an extra loop of fabric is put there for that purpose.

Wallets

Replace your old wallet before it begins to look shabby. Good leather absorbs a lot of wear, but eventually it has had its day. If you have one of those canvas and Velcro types of wallet, it is ready for replacement, no matter how old.

Select a slim, all-leather wallet in brown or black, devoid of any embellishment or adornment. Do not overfill it to the point of stretching the leather or creating a bulge in the line of your trousers. If you carry more cards and papers than will fit easily in your wallet, consider the breast-pocket type of wallet known as a secretary. Secretary-type billfolds have an undisputed aura of elegance.

Briefcases

As with your wallet, your briefcase should be leather. Your choice of color extends to the various shades of brown; black is regarded as unseemly. Brass clasps and a plain leather handle are standard good form. Any unusual stitching, materials, or markings detract from their effect.

A rectangular, full-sized attaché case is often more practical than a slim model or a leather envelope-type case. It can double as the smallest of suitcases and hold a clean shirt. But any of the three styles is perfectly acceptable in all business circles. Questioning glances, however, greet shoulder bags: A handle, not a strap, is what your case should have.

Umbrellas

Umbrellas should be black, folding or straight, and traditional in appearance when opened. There is very little deviant opinion about umbrellas—except as to why it is the human condition to keep the $6 one for years and lose the $30 one the first time you use it.

14

The *Dress for Excellence* Travel Adviser

The Geography of Power

Wherever you go in the United States, men who are at the top dress pretty much the same way. They buy expensive clothes, their accessories are impeccable, and they enjoy looking good.

At the same time, there are differences. Just as men in the North and Northeast dress in lighter colors in summer months and in darker colors during the winter, so, too, do men dress somewhat differently depending upon geography. In warmer climates, clothes tend to be a bit lighter—both in weight and color—all year round. But only a little. As any well-dressed southerner will tell you, "Only the tourists wear white in winter."

177

A few other characteristic differences:

- **California** isn't just one state; for visiting businessmen it is two distinct regions. Studiedly casual clothes are worn in Los Angeles, especially by top people in the film and television industries. You will notice on the one hand more freedom, even jeans without jackets (a casual look that may be "finished" by an expensively tailored shirt). Yet you can scarcely find a more traditional group of businessmen than those in the downtown Los Angeles financial district. In the best restaurants you will observe conservative suits in boardroom blue and bankers' gray.

  San Francisco architects, bankers, high-tech executives, and lawyers are all business. The Brooks Brothers style of dressing looms large here. Because of the cool summers, men in San Francisco tend to wear the same traditional clothes most of the year.

- In **Texas** successful businessmen really do wear western hats and expensive boots—often with conservatively cut Ivy League suits. But visiting easterners should not try to affect this look.

- **Kansas** and the Plains States are scorching in summer and bone-chillingly frigid in winter. The lightest-weight wools or poplins will fill the bill if you travel there in July and August; a suede, shearling-lined top coat is a smart idea from November through March.

- Abrupt changes in the weather are commonplace in **Oregon and Washington.** When visiting the region, a Gore-Tex® featherweight parka shell can be the handiest item in your flight bag. It repels rain and protects you from out-of-season snow flurries. Although it should not be worn over business suits, it can be worn on weekends—and is perfect for plant visits in rough weather.

- **Miami**'s nearly total climate control—air-conditioning in every conceivable structure—has changed the way Miamians dress. Cotton cords, poplins, and Palm Beach suits are no longer necessary. Outwardly, a southern Florida businessman resembles the branch managers of his firm in Chicago and Washington.

  The March 24, 1985, issue of *The New York Times Magazine*'s authoritative style roundup, "Men's Fashions of the Times," carried an article on business attire around the country. From it, I noted what works in several major cities.

- In **Washington,** the lawyer, the lobbyist, the corporate executive, and the Foreign Service officer all favor sober dark suits at all times of the year. But every Washington male has at least one khaki or seersucker suit in his wardrobe for the dregs of August.
- **Denver**'s oilmen share the cowboy boot and the Stetson with the stockmen, but take the rest of their cues from Houston and Dallas. This means wearing two-piece suits.
- **Atlanta** remains a stronghold of the traditionalist. For out-of-towners, the best advice is: Go conservative. Remember that Atlanta's idea of a trendy look is a bow tie, suspenders, and a shirt with a plain point collar.
- The **Boston** businessman considers his dark suit, white shirt, and red tie to be virtually a uniform. Chances are that he whose suit has padded shoulders and pleated slacks owns his own business.

Are There Regional Differences in Men's Dress?

Oh, sure. In a town of 100,000, I have gotten in the habit of wearing sportscoats. It's a combination of the size of the city, the South, and the heat in the summer. But when I go to Atlanta or Chicago, I wear a suit.

Overdressing tells you a lot. Chances are a good line of blather goes with it. If someone appears in Albany, Georgia, too flashily dressed, well . . .

—JAMES C. MAINWOOD,
president,
Lilliston Corporation,
farm equipment manufacturers,
Albany, Georgia

New York—Not So Different

New Yorkers dress in classic business clothes during business hours. Every hint, tip, rule, and chart about office dressing you've read in these pages is pertinent to the New York mode.

After-office dressing in New York is, of course, quite different. In Manhattan the very best East Side restaurants assume that their guests will follow accepted dress codes. Popular restaurants and bars in SoHo and on the Upper West Side most emphatically do not make that assumption.

Yet I have begun to see top men on Wall Street, whom the rest of the country's financial people try to emulate by dressing ultraconservatively, starting to experiment with eclectic dressing. Certainly not all, or even a high percentage of them do this. But suits with pleated trousers, subtly padded shoulders, and double-breasted silhouettes; slightly shorter shirt collars; smaller necktie knots—all these are modifying the traditional Wall Street look among a few avant-garde executives.

Wrinkle-Free Packing
for Wherever Life Takes You

Somewhere between the extremes of packing too much or too little is the right formula for travel. If a man were to wear a blazer on the plane, pack two suits, three shirts, and four ties, his appearance during a three-day trip would improve tremendously. But if you cannot carry the extra suit, at least put in one extra shirt and two or three extra ties. They take very little room and increase your options significantly. If one of your shirts loses a button and one of your ties gets spotted, why be down to a perilous minimum?

When packing your suitcase, never leave empty space. The extra room allows your clothes to move about and become wrinkled. Either use a smaller bag or fill the one you have with plastic dry cleaner's bags.

Here is the secret to wrinkle-free packing: When your clothes come from the cleaner's, keep them in those thin plastic bags. Let them remain in the bags, on the hangers, and with all of the tissue paper stuffing the cleaner puts in the shoulders. Put the whole works into your suitcase, either a conventional suitcase (I'll tell you how to fold the jacket in a moment), or a hanging garment bag, which I prefer. With plastic covers between the items, your clothes are protected from rubbing against each other and will not wrinkle. Even with the huge number of clothes that I take on my trips—both my own clothing and the men's clothes that I show in my programs—everything gets there wrinkle-free if I pack rather full and use plastic garment bags.

Taking this plastic trick one step further, you can use extra plastic bags as insulators between items to give you double protection from wrinkles. Despite these precautions, something may need ironing when you arrive at a hotel. The valet or bellman should be at your door to pick it up in ten minutes. If there is a significant delay, or if you need the clothing immediately, phone the housekeeping department for an iron and ironing board. Every hotel has them. The big, new hotel chains generally tell you that they have two irons for 1,500 rooms and that both are being used. Insist firmly and relentlessly. Miraculously an iron will materialize.

Easier to use than an iron, if you can locate one, is a little hand-held steamer. You simply fill it with water, plug it in, and pass it back and forth *near* the wrinkles. It is a great invention, and will remove any unexpected wrinkle that creeps into a suit jacket.

Without an iron or a steamer, you still have one last resort. Take the wrinkled item out of the plastic bag, but leave it on the hanger. Put it in the bathroom—hang it as high as possible, not too near the shower—and turn on the hot water. Close the bathroom door and allow steam to fill the room for about ten minutes. The wrinkles will disappear, especially from woolen clothes. Allow time for the garment to cool before you wear it, or you will wrinkle it anew.

If you do not hang your clothes in a garment bag, but prefer the flat-pack method, pack your jacket as follows: Fold the jacket in half lengthwise with the two lapels facing out. Put your hand inside one shoulder, and fold the other shoulder around it so that the outer one is now inside out. If your suitcase is large enough to lay this out flat, do so. If it will not fit, then place either a plastic bag or a few sheets of tissue paper (saved from shopping trips) over it and fold the jacket in half. The process is easier done than described.

Some fastidious men have all their shirts ironed at the laundry and delivered on hangers. These same men usually have a few of their shirts folded at the laundry for easier packing when going on trips. If you are using a garment bag, I suggest you still have your shirts hung on hangers; it is a cinch to slip them into the bag.

A Guide to Fine Shopping
Away from Home

Certainly work will take up the lion's share of your time when you travel on business. But one of the pleasures of going to new places is the wealth of wonderful stores to explore. I urge you to visit some of these superior ones in selected cities.

ATLANTA	Britches of Georgetowne, Davison's, Mark Shale, George Muse, Neiman-Marcus, Rich's
BALTIMORE	Hutzler's, Eddie Jacobs
BOSTON	Jordan Marsh, Louis, J. Press, Roots, W. D. and Company
CHARLOTTE	Jodphur's
CHICAGO	Bigsby & Kruthers, Brittany Ltd., Mark Shale, Marshall Field, Neiman-Marcus, Ultimo Ltd.
COLUMBUS	Lazarus
DALLAS	Arresta, Clyde Campbell, Harold's, Mark Shale, Neiman-Marcus, Outfitters, Sanger Harris
DENVER	Perkins Shearer
HOUSTON	Frost Brothers, Neiman-Marcus, Sakowitz
KANSAS CITY	Mr. Guy, Saks Fifth Avenue, Woolf Brothers
LOS ANGELES	Bijan, Bullock's Wilshire, Giorgio, Jerry Magnin, Maxfield, Neiman-Marcus, Perkins Shearer
MIAMI	Burdine's, Raphael, The Twenty-Four Collection
MINNEAPOLIS	The Dayton Company
NEW ORLEANS	Porter Stevens, Rubenstein Bros., Weinstein's
NEW YORK CITY	Andre Oliver, Barneys, Bergdorf Goodman, Brioni, Alfred Dunhill, Bloomingdale's, Bonwit Teller, Brooks Brothers, Hermès, Lord & Taylor, Paul Stuart, Polo/Ralph Lauren, J. Press, Sulka, F. R. Tripler & Co.

OKLAHOMA CITY	Cappuccio, Harold's
PHILADELPHIA	Boyd's Gushner, Dimensions, John Wanamaker
PITTSBURGH	Joseph Horne, Larrimor's
PORTLAND	Mario's
SAN FRANCISCO	I. Magnin, J. Press, Wilkes Bashford
SEATTLE	Frederick & Nelson, Nordstrom
WASHINGTON, D.C.	Arthur Adler, Britches of Georgetowne, Garfinckel's, Raleigh's, Woodward & Lothrop

The Vital Carry-On Bag

When shopping for an underseat carry-on bag, choose a zippered one that is roomy yet still able to fit easily under a plane seat. Be extremely cautious that it doesn't exceed the airlines' allowable size limit: length, width, and breadth cannot total more than forty-four inches.

Heavy leather luggage is prestigious (or used to be, when skycaps were plentiful), but it is also a ball and chain when you are dashing through miles of airport corridors with only minutes to spare. Go for stylish, lightweight nylon or canvas, and choose one of the reputable, well-constructed brands. As in most instances, pay a little more and you'll have a handsome bag that will stay handsome.

The longer your trip, the more important are the items that travel with you in your carry-on bag. Your checked-on suitcase may wind up in Tulsa, but your hand is firmly on your carry-on bag as you deplane in Houston, and in it are these necessities:

· **Toiletry kit.** To lose it would be a catastrophe. Even if leaks occur, your suits and ties won't be ruined, since they are packed in the garment bag or suitcase. Cut down possible damage to the other contents of your carry-on bag by enclosing your toilet kit in one of those handy zip-locked plastic bags. And don't forget to slip any necessary medications into your kit.

· **Extra shirt and tie.** What is the minimum clothing needed to save you at tomorrow's meeting if the airline loses your suitcase today? You can squeak through with a change of shirt and tie. Pack one of each in your carry-on bag. Choose a wrinkle-free cotton/polyester blend for the shirt, and a silk tie wrapped in several layers of tissue.

· **Sweater, cap, and gloves.** Between airport, airplane, outdoors, and hotel, temperatures can range from stuffy and hot to chilly or freezing. If your suitcase is delayed or lost, these items will be lifesavers during your stay.

· **Pen, paper, and important documents.** Although the props I use in my sessions are checked through, I always have an extra set of notes in my carry-on bag. If the airline should lose my luggage and I have to present a program without visuals, the extra set of notes is my "security blanket" if it becomes necessary to wing it.

I don't use expensive luggage with elaborate locks. To do so would be to wave a flag and announce that what's inside is valuable. Status luggage is fine for your carry-on piece, but select something innocuous for checking.

15

Perfecting Your Personal Style

Your Reasons for a Personal Style

The power of personal style was illustrated to me perfectly one evening in Indianapolis. I was working with several managers of the J I Case Company to set up a presentation for a meeting I was addressing the next day. It was late when we were through, and we went down to the hotel bar to relax.

When the waitress brought our bill, she never asked who was paying. She just put it down in front of the right man, the ranking officer. How did she know? He was wearing a blazer and a handsome, vivid blue tie—an unusual tie, but he wore it with aplomb and confidence. His looks said, "I'm in charge."

The manager—I'll call him Ed—is no exhibitionist. But he enjoys being noticed and remembered. His image has been perked up with the dash and flair that accrue to those who make good use of a distinctive element or style in dress.

There are several reasons why a successful man will adopt a singular style or "trademark" item of clothing. It may make him stand out from the crowd or express an aspect of his personality that he feels merits public attention. Or he may simply like the way it makes him look.

Ed's tie worked well for him, but not everyone would be comfortable making such a singular statement. A much easier approach would be immersion in one mode of dress. It could be a Brooks Brothers look— one so complete that you'd think the wearer stepped off the pages of the latest Brooks catalog—or it could be a vigorous pursuit of the impeccable Wall Street look.

Go Slowly

To start expressing your personal style—and I'll describe at least twenty ways other managers are doing it—do it quietly. Begin slowly, with quiet points of difference. One way to break out while staying within your company's dress requirements (if they are very conservative) is to wear subtly patterned socks.

Here are a number of other subtle touches of individualism I have noticed among executives. One of them might be closely attuned to your image of yourself.

- Carry a fine, imported leather briefcase.
- Enjoy the tactile pleasure of carrying the finest alligator wallet and wearing a beautifully made alligator belt.
- Your quiet point of distinction may come from wearing pleated trousers with your traditionally cut suits.
- Although everyone around you wears button-down shirts, yours may have beautifully laundered point collars, worn with a collar pin.
- A made-to-measure shirt gives you the confidence that comes of knowing you feel comfortable and look impeccable. You may find that colored shirts look interesting on your colleagues, but that you enjoy consistently wearing crisp, white, flawlessly fitting ones.

An Outside Chance

You may be constrained by company disapproval of deviations from "accepted" office dress. Outerwear, donned as you head for the elevators, may be the answer.

How about an Irish tweed hat . . . or a classic fedora?

Or a white cashmere scarf . . . or a long, brightly colored muffler?

Or the finest leather gloves you can buy—the kind that can be tucked in your topcoat's breast pocket?

- You might collect antique cuff links and wear them in your French-cuffed shirts.
- Consider growing a mustache as a fine focal point. An uncommon but modest pair of eyeglasses may accomplish the same purpose.
- Personalize your wardrobe with color, emphasizing one or two shades in which you look your best and often get compliments.
- Regularly wear the finest shoes you can afford. They will be made of the most supple leather, several cuts above the footwear of your colleagues. (Will they know? Maybe not, but you will.)
- Become a regular client of the best hair stylist in town. Women are still in their teens when they realize they're not at their best unless their hair is exactly right. Too many men never learn this lesson, and give themselves a handicap.
- There's the old reliable: a pocket square or linen handkerchief in your breast pocket.

Any of these suggestions is the sort of touch that still leaves you well within the confines of codes for conventional dressing. Not one of them says, "He's trying too hard; he looks like a fashion plate."

So long as you adopt only one or two of these or similar touches, you are gaining distinction. But if you were to incorporate several, the effect would be counterproductive. You would be seen as being too concerned with yourself and your looks.

> When you break one rule, deliberately and elegantly, that is dressing with distinction. When you break several, you are seen as a person who just doesn't know the rules.

A Variety of Touches

Proceeding from the subtle to the more noticeable, many new possibilities arise.

- Wear a bow tie.
- Wear only one kind of necktie—Hermès would be a prime choice—and own enough of them so you needn't vary from your custom.
- Carry a pocket watch instead of wearing a wristwatch. Perhaps it is one your father or grandfather wore. Or you might purchase an antique that's not pretentious or large, and wear it on a chain.
- Wear a new fashion-forward suit, one with a nonvented jacket and pleated trousers.
- Wear a double-breasted suit.
- Try a shirt with a colored or striped body and a white contrast collar.
- Wear noticeably well-coordinated neckties and suspenders. One set might include a yellow background foulard tie and blue, yellow, and pink striped suspenders, worn on a white or blue shirt.
- Be true to your tweedy personality, if that's "really you." Go for argyle sweaters and a pipe, and don't be seen in pin-striped suits.
- Make a personality statement by wearing a strongly colored necktie. It might be medium blue with widely spaced khaki stripes, perfect with your tan summer suit.
- Be a "sweater man," collecting as many styles and colors as you can for wear with blazers and weekend dressing.
- Try the new, lower cut loafers that expose more of your sock, and introduce some understated patterns into your sock wardrobe.

When a frankly flamboyant touch is adopted as a man's "signature" item—Van Johnson's celebrated fire-engine red socks come to mind—many might consider it just this side of eccentricity. A boutonnière adds dash and verve to a confident man's appearance, but not everyone would choose a flower worn on the lapel as his signature look. Franklin Roosevelt wore a cape and brandished a long cigarette holder; he was able to assimilate those showy touches into his intense personal style. They complemented his aristocratic bearing; for FDR, they were credible mannerisms.

Not everyone need make an effort to be noticed. If being a standout is the path for you, fine, as long as you exercise restraint. Don't risk being thought an exhibitionist.

> I asked Stanley Marcus if he thought a man had leeway to dress less conservatively as he moved up the ladder of success. I mentioned FDR's cape as one outstanding departure from the rules. He answered, "Position and age—both youth and seniority—endow a man with a certain degree of daring. A young blade may wear an evening cape because he wants to startle people. An older man may wear one because he doesn't give a damn."

Colors Project Your Personality

You know that certain suit colors—dark blue with pinstripes, particularly—reflect authority and power. Others, notably tan and medium blues, suggest the facilitator, the person whose approach is "let's work together."

You can use this knowledge to build a personal style. If you want to be welcomed, accepted by men (and women), wear what I call "love me" colors: ones that carry no threat. Cream-colored shirts, gray stripes on white, red and white stripes that meld into pink—all these may ease your acceptance into circles where you are unknown or at times when you are still sizing up a situation and are not yet ready to make an unequivocal personal statement.

Be aware, though, that while a tan *suit* sends out a message about facilitating, a heavily tanned *complexion* impresses most observers as a power statement. Having a tan implies that you have the leisure to acquire one. It also casts an aura of good health and peak condition.

Blue and white stripes of a conventional hue in a traditional oxford cloth, Ivy League shirt can be seen and not noticed. But for distinction, try a smooth-surfaced broadcloth white shirt with bold blue stripes. The bolder the stripes, the wider the spacing, and the more intense the shade of blue, the more powerful the statement. Try Bengal stripes, which are thin but narrowly and evenly spaced, and are at their best when woven of dark blue or burgundy threads. Worn with a light tan summer suit of gabardine or poplin, the effect is one of sophistication and power.

Fitness and Grooming

The Shape You're In

Exercise, goes the old wheeze, is what you needed yesterday and are going to start tomorrow. Today, increasing numbers of men realize the benefits of a well-conditioned body.

Your clothes cannot disguise a general lack of body tone, a tendency toward flab rather than firmness, and a lack of vitality. Daily walking, running, swimming, or a fifteen-minute regimen of carefully planned exercise is so essential that I assume you have already chosen your own routine.

I wish I could remember the name of the brilliant doctor—I think he was a cardiologist—who advised a person who has only one hour to spend and wants to know the safest way to spend it. "Lie down and do nothing," he said. "But if a person has a lifetime to spend, he shouldn't spend that hour sitting; he'd be much better off exercising."

Part of looking good is not just exercising, but having a diet that gives you the energy you need to fulfill your goals. The evidence is overwhelming that cigarette smoking, being dangerously overweight, and a high cholesterol diet are associated with a host of health problems.

According to Howard R. Sloan, M.D., Ph.D., head of the Division of Biochemical Disorders at Ohio State University's College of Medicine,

"The American Heart Association's prudent diet suggests that no one consume more than 300 milligrams of cholesterol per day. Unfortunately, one egg contains 300 milligrams of cholesterol, so that one would not be able to eat any other animal product that day and still keep within the suggested guidelines." Of course you will have days when it is difficult to stick to the ideal of what is best for you, but always be aware that what you put into your body directly influences your effectiveness as a leader.

Think of the executives you know whose smiles are important focal points of their notable appearances. They treasure and preserve their teeth. Perhaps doing this costs more than a tie or blazer, but the effect is worth it.

Commit Yourself to Proper Dental Care

For you, the first step is to realize the admiration you will attract with white, even teeth. Once you are aware of any gaps, discoloration, or chips that flaw your smile, you can have them remedied.

One serious flaw that you may not discern in the mirror is bad breath. That can be a serious handicap at work, as well as devastating to your social life—because you don't know if you have the problem. But everyone else does! My guess is that if you are a heavy smoker, you can be sure you do. Brush your teeth more often and use a mouthwash. It should lessen the problem.

Decay, the cause of most mouth odors, can be located and eradicated by any dental general practitioner.

Dentists can work miracles. New bonding techniques, in which layers of acrylic are applied to existing teeth to fill gaps and chips, are painless. They are done fairly quickly, with no more than an hour per tooth required for normal sessions.

Norman Trieger, D.M.D., M.D., and chairman of the Department of Dentistry at Montefiore Medical Center in New York, told me how often he is surprised to meet a man wearing an $800 suit whose teeth are decayed, crooked, or missing. "It certainly has nothing to do with the cost of dental treatment," he said. "They are walking around like that because of their tremendous fear of dental work." New techniques and anti-anxiety medications make those fears groundless, he told me. The patient remains awake through the whole procedure and has little or no discomfort.

Dr. Trieger mentioned that the incidence of decay is higher in New

England and the Deep South than in other parts of the country. People of Scottish and Irish descent have inherently lower resistance to decay.

He has found that lack of proper dental care and the passing of years are responsible for diminished attractiveness in some men's faces. Before it becomes noticeable and distracting, corrective dentistry is a must. Years of wear and tear on teeth cause jaw muscles to expand. The face loses its vertical aspect, the chin becomes prominent, the edges of the mouth turn down, and increasingly fewer teeth are visible. Dentists today have techniques for building up and restoring the bite, and in that way restoring the height of the face.

Several trips to the dentist each year for thorough cleaning and inspection should deter problems. And the twice-a-day brushing that was urged on you in grade school is a habit you were wise to retain. Flossing between the teeth is added protection. The gleam of well-conditioned teeth you'll flash when you smile is worth the extra minute or two it takes to achieve it.

Your Hair

Just as you made it clear to the salesman and tailor that you are in charge of your appearance, so you will want to have a similar relationship with your barber. Once a month you are putting a key aspect of your appearance in his hands. He is skilled in his trade, and you value his advice. But you must make the decisions, and your haircut should proceed unhurriedly to exactly the finish that you have described.

Once you have arrived at the style that's best for you, and you know that this barber is capable of achieving it, stay with him. "Just like last time" is what he has to hear, and a reminder of last time's special points: not close over here, a little bit longer here and here, and don't touch the top. You're in his hands, but you're watching carefully in the mirror. And in his hand, when he's done that perfect job, goes a tip generous enough—about 20 percent—to guarantee he *will* remember you next month.

Of all the hairstyles available to you, your choice will depend on two factors. The first is the general image you want to convey. It might be young, fashion-forward, and very much with the current trend. It might be conservative: the hairstyle that senior executives have retained for decades past and will be wearing for decades to come. Or it might be slightly dashing—not theatrical or extreme, but a trifle more commanding of attention than the usual.

The other factor is the natural one: the color and thickness of your hair, its curliness or straightness, and most especially the shape of your head and face. Work with what you have. You can lengthen a round face by adding some height to the top of your head. Or if your face is thin, who had a thinner one than dapper Fred Astaire? He slicked his hair down as close to the scalp as possible, allowing no more height to an already vertical face.

Don't worry about shampooing your hair too frequently. If you are not genetically disposed toward baldness, you can wash your hair as often as is necessary for a neat appearance. If you are balding, and you care about it, you should gently wash your hair *daily* with a mild shampoo.

Persistent dryness can lead to hair damage. Even more damaging is the harsh, astringent action of ordinary soap. If you have problems with your hair or scalp, a good shampoo recommended by a reliable pharmacist (or a dermatologist, if you consult one) is a necessity.

Using a conditioner or one of the newer products such as a controlling mousse will allow you to maintain all day the hairstyle that you saw in your bathroom mirror this morning. It also will give a fuller look to your hair. You may prefer the old-fashioned "little dab" of your favorite hair-grooming product. Whichever you choose, use slightly less than the instructions on the label direct you to use; a very little dab will do it.

If you are bald, or are losing hair rapidly, in all likelihood you have consulted a doctor about it. But I would like to stress that *the only people who are turned off by baldness are the owners of the bald heads themselves.* Most people don't care whether you are balding or not. It is not a deterrent to business or social success. When I was a freshman in college, there was one fellow, a senior, who was bald. All of the girls thought he was the sexiest guy around.

If you wear a beard or a mustache, go on occasion to one of the finest barbershops. See how he trims and grooms it. When at home, simply follow his lines. Any style that is not too exaggerated and that pleases you is the right style *if* you don't allow it to become scraggly.

Your Hands

Your hands are always on display, and fingernails tell a lot about a person. Don't ignore them. A business or professional man has no excuse for hands and nails that look less than perfect.

Nails look their best when kept all the same length—short—and scrubbed clean. All the equipment you need is a pair of clippers and a nailbrush. Bitten nails tell people you are nervous and not in control. They are guaranteed to detract from an executive's image.

I recommend an occasional manicure just so you can see how short to clip your nails, how far to push back your cuticles, and how good your hands can look. However, do not under any circumstances allow anyone to put polish on your nails. Even clear nail polish has a negative connotation.

Business Scents

In the same way that smoking assaults many people's sensitivities, so does too much cologne.

One way to tell if your scent choice is the best one for you is by learning what others think about it. Listen for, "You smell so great today," or "I like your after-shave."

More important than the scent itself is the intensity. After-shave, which is lighter than cologne and more of a skin-treatment product than a scent, is fine for an office setting. Reserve cologne, which is stronger, for evening, social situations.

In my opinion, unless you are dancing with someone (or are closer to a person than is appropriate in business), you should not be able to detect a scent.

Body Odor

A tennis court or locker room is the only place where body odor is acceptable—and then only until the offending person reaches the showers. Deodorant soaps for all-over help; drying yourself thoroughly; using antiperspirants, spray or roll-on deodorants, and talcum powder for those parts of the body where you can't use deodorant—all work.

Stressful situations can increase perspiration and necessitate stronger measures. Between showers, splash quickly and rewash underarms to freshen your body, or use a small roll-on kept in your desk—you'll feel better. Wearing cotton T-shirts and all-cotton shirts also helps. Synthetic fabrics are notorious for increasing perspiration and retaining odor.

To avoid any problems with foot odor, wear natural-fiber (cotton or wool) socks; they absorb perspiration better than synthetic ones. Foot powders also help to keep the feet dry.

Most women agree that the most attractive odor a man can have is a clean, freshly scrubbed natural smell, maintained with the help of a deodorant.

Coping with Success

Establishing an enviable personal style; attracting favorable notice in corporate corridors; feeling fit and looking it: These things are yours to claim. And I believe they aren't exactly new to you; you've had your share of success.

Yet I hope you've made a note, as you read this chapter, to try a new tack or two. Maybe you will be a shade more daring in your choice of hat. Perhaps your teeth will gleam more intensely, or your hair reflect a new vitality. Well, I say this is exactly the time for it. Because in the next chapter you'll learn my formula for dressing to appeal to women. Grooming and flair count plenty with women, and so do the tips you'll accumulate which follow.

16

Dressing to Appeal to Women

If it is true that "power is the ultimate aphrodisiac" for men, it is no less so for women. Think of the many famous men who are not everyone's idea of handsome, yet who attract the world's most desirable women. I'm convinced that the look of power is a look that women find immensely appealing. Everything that assures your recognition in the office works equally well in a man-woman relationship.

Today's confident woman wants to know that her man is worthy of her esteem and is as capable as she is of taking charge. She would like to know that he can do what's necessary if unexpected, unpleasant circumstances crop up—and what's necessary in the delightfully pleasant circumstances that she anticipates. She would like to feel that people who meet them recognize her man as a person of assurance and consequence.

Can clothes do all this? No; it would be foolish to imply that people are impressionable to that degree. Yet, as I have mentioned before, at first glance they have no other way of assessing a person's character. They make snap decisions about his professional, social, and sexual desirability and so they base their impressions on the only evidence they see: his appearance.

In a room filled with people, in your own or in her office; in a restaurant or on a plane—wherever you are introduced to a discerning woman, she will be attracted to the man who reflects confidence, flair, and a strong sense of his own worth.

The Look That Attracts Women

· **Complementary.** Women appreciate being appreciated. And one of the most obvious ways for a man to show his regard is to dress in a mode that is compatible with hers. If a man and a woman are going to the theater, a good restaurant, or an event he knows will prompt her to dress to the nines, he should dress accordingly. To wear a plaid or a tweed sportscoat and an open-neck shirt is a not-so-subtle form of disregard. It betrays a self-absorption that leaves no room for others.

The trait that will guarantee your appearance to complement a woman's is *consideration*. And nothing, I assure you, rates higher on

---

The actress Sally Field was quoted in a *People* interview ("The Man Is Back," by Jane Hall, *People,* Apr. 22, 1985) about James Garner, her leading man in the movie *Murphy's Romance*. "If men only knew," sighed Field. "What's appealing to a woman is how a man makes her feel about herself. Jim is funny and dear, and he laughs at my jokes. That's what makes Jim sexy; it doesn't change with years."

most women's "wanted" lists than a man who is considerate. Just do this: Before reaching into the closet for the outfit that suits your whim, think of what *she* will be wearing. Then consider what you can wear that will set it off—complement it—in the way she'll find most gratifying.

In this instance, virtue is doubly rewarded. You will have her appreciation, even admiration, and your own appearance will be enhanced. After all, you're half of that striking couple.

· **Flair.** Ask any fisherman: Lively bait gets bitten at. And although I see little similarity between Ms. Smith, the investment counselor at First National, and a speckled trout, I do know that both are attracted by a flash of sparkle and color.

When women dress well, their aim is to leave the mundane back there in the closet. They are attracted to a man who does the same, but without abandoning the subtlety and understatement that I advocate so often in this book.

Try several of the suggestions in chapter 15, "Perfecting Your Personal Style." Or wear a yellow tie with your dark gray suit, rather than the expected blue or burgundy one. Or show up wearing the snap-brim felt hat that Stetson has never stopped manufacturing and dapper men have never stopped wearing. Try a tab-collared shirt or one with a white contrast collar; or a silk tie with an all-over paisley pattern in muted red.

In your choice of shirts, sweaters, and pants for casual wear, you might move toward somewhat lighter and brighter shades. A sweater that is off-white instead of beige—or even one that is periwinkle (a light blue that leans toward lavender) instead of medium blue—might elicit a whole new reaction when seen through feminine eyes. In the same way, keep an open mind about coral or tangerine as polo shirt colors, rather than sticking with the fireman's red that has seen you through so many seasons of casual wear.

When I see a sophisticated dresser with a bit of dash about him, I'm inclined to think, "How clever of him. I'll bet he'd be fun to talk to." And like any human being, I nudge the laws of circumstance and coincidence a little, so that we *do* talk.

· **Restraint.** Most women are attracted to fit men who have tanned, healthy skin tones. Except at the beach or at a pool, however, they consider it inappropriate for a man to flaunt his body.

Shirts open to the navel or sleeves rolled up to the shoulder are immediate turnoffs to any woman of style and taste. To her, supermacho is crude and uninviting.

In only one instance would I advocate less restraint and more flesh, and that's where Bermuda shorts are concerned. These "gentlemanly" shorts look affected on any but the most British dressers. Regular-length shorts—the kind you'd wear for tennis or volleyball—are much preferred. They're straightforward—and if you have the legs for them, flaunt them.

· **Details.** Women notice a sloppy ironing job (as they are often too well acquainted with ironing); frayed shirt cuffs; perspiration discoloration on shirts or coats; scuffed shoes; a badly trimmed mustache (they can *feel* this one, too); sagging socks.

And they are as quick to notice attractive details: fine leather accessories; simple but elegant cuff links; a blue shirt that matches your eyes; an impressive cashmere scarf.

In *Hard Money,* a fine novel by Michael M. Thomas (Viking Penguin Inc., 1985), the narrator recalls the dress sense of a celebrated communications tycoon whose appeal to women was legendary.

". . . a soft dark-gray suit, one of probably fifty; a shirt patterned in minute blue checks, the collar latched under the small knot of a navy blue knitted silk necktie by a gold safety pin; dark brown slip-on shoes polished to a mirrorlike gleam . . . Keep it simple, boys, he used to tell Abner and me. Don't dress like a salesman: no Windsor knots, no patterns in the suiting. Being classy's nine tenths a matter of discretion."

· **Quality.** Most women know more about fabrics and tailoring than do most men. They recognize fine materials and first-class workmanship in a suit as well as a dress, and they are aware of the cost. A man who has self-esteem enough to spend whatever it costs—and she knows it costs plenty—to look exactly right is a man who gains an extra measure of her admiration.

Take the small matter of gloves. Any woman with a sense of fashion can distinguish between a pair of stiff leather gloves that cost $14.95 and

a luxuriously soft, lined-with-cashmere pair that costs $50. I'm not sug-
gesting that you try to buy esteem, or that a woman who has a mind
attuned to cash registers is estimable. Rather, I am restating a point that
cannot be overemphasized: *Go for the best.* Your credentials will be
established on first sight.

· **Fit,** in both senses of the word. Women are attracted to a man who
is fit and well groomed and whose clothes fit with flattering precision.

The impressions that hair, skin, scent, and other aspects of grooming
make on business associates were discussed in the preceding chapter. For
all the reasons stated there, you will want to keep your body—the
essential *you*—as alluring as you can. (Did you know that the turnoff
most consistently mentioned by women is dirty fingernails?) Only the
most naive of men can be unconcerned about the effect on women of
their physical features, and particularly of scent.

Some years ago, I was determined to learn, from as many women as I
could, what kinds of cologne attracted or repelled them. I talked to forty
or fifty women who were representative of women likely to have social
contact with readers of this book. They were practically unanimous in
their dislike of overly strong "heavy" colognes. What they like are
straight after-shaves and light colognes, ones that "aren't fancy," ones
that "smell like my dad." Not knowing what their dads were like, I
translate that as masculine but not overpowering. Eau Sauvage (by Chris-
tian Dior) and Paco Rabanne were the two brands most mentioned, and
several of the more sophisticated women said that *vetiver,* an aroma
pressed from European and Asian herbs, is irresistible.

Beyond Your Appearance

Women respond to courtesy and respect. They accept—more often, they
demand—the new "courtesies" of the 1980s: independence, equality, and
a parallel lane on the fast track. But they see no conflict between those
requisites and a man's ability to treat them as if they were *women.* That
has nothing to do with who picks up the check or holds open the door.

It has everything to do with an attitude, a general demeanor, that
women can sense immediately.

One woman I talked with made an intriguing comment. "I think the
men I really respond to are ones who have a sister at home. They know

how to treat women. They may take them for granted at times, yet right there, up on top, is respect. And love; they're capable of love."

If you value the uniqueness of the woman in your life, you can be sure she will discern your feelings. Your appreciation of her will be apparent, just as your appreciation of your own worth is apparent in your determination to enhance your image. People respond to a drive for excellence. Whether it is called "dressing for business" or "dressing for women," the end result is heightened self-esteem and heightened appeal to others. You'll find them both most gratifying.

17

Dressing for Power
Away from
the Office

In the world of business not every day is nine to five. Some mornings begin with a 7:30 breakfast meeting. Some involve formal business lunches. Other days a field trip to a plant may dominate your schedule, or they may involve a 6 A.M. tennis game or a round of after-work golf where more deals may be initiated than in three months of office groundwork.

On some days, you go directly from work for drinks with colleagues. And, when you are one of the chosen few, you might fly away to a sparkling resort for a three-day conference. All of this is business. It just doesn't happen to occur in the office.

Your clothes continue to express your personality and position, even in nonwork situations, but often it is more difficult to know what to wear for these semisocial, semiwork occasions than for the regular workaday world. And the further you advance up the ladder, the more often these situations arise.

Each time, the main concern is professionalism, comfort, appropriateness, and good looks. Haphazard selections won't do.

The Wonderful World of Almost-Fashion

These are the perfect times to try some selections from the wonderful world of advancing fashion displayed in magazines and in the stores, provided you don't go overboard. Blazers, pleated trousers, cashmere sweaters, flannel shirts, rugby shirts, loafers, topsiders, New Wave black-tie dressing, perhaps even a silk shirt or an ultrasuede jacket can fit some of the times when business and social life overlap. Keep in mind that there's no good time for looking bad, and no bad time for looking good.

FRIDAY:
Dressing for Friday

In many work situations, people dress differently on Fridays from the way they do on the other days of the week. The idea is partly image: You want to show that you have an outside life. Dressing differently on Friday implies an upcoming weekend. It also can indicate success. It may suggest, for example, that you are leaving work to go to your country house. Maybe you're only going to Grandma's. But dressing down a bit shows a touch of independence and implies a weekend of leisure.

A wise procedure is to try not to schedule a major formal conference on Friday so that you can dress a bit more casually. Wear a tweed jacket in winter—or a blazer, which works well any time of the year. They are great with a button-down dress shirt, a casual tie of wool knit or linen, loafers, and a slightly avant-garde pair of trousers, perhaps with pleats (a good way to update your look). The sexy tight-jeans look of yesteryear is passé. As with women's sweaters, the less body shown, the more interesting the body.

This more casual Friday outfit is useful for other occasions, too: fieldwork, a plant visit, a rainy, miserable day—all so long as you are *not* breaking company guidelines. In many conservatively structured companies, you don't have a casual dress option, Friday or not. In such cases, your way of expressing your success and conveying the healthy impression of having a life outside work may be by bringing your weekend duffel bag to the office. A man in my audience once asked me, "What do you think I should do? My boss insists that we wear dark suits and ties every day. He is adamant against blazers in the office, even on Fridays." My answer was, "If your boss really is adamant against blazers, I think you should wear a suit every day." That didn't take a great deal of insight—the boss *is* the boss.

SATURDAY:
Working on a Nonworkday
(That was a short weekend!)

Although you are coming in to work on a Saturday, your attire should reinforce the fact that you know it is the weekend and don't feel that life is all work.

Let the circumstances dictate your appearance. Does the company have a strict policy about dress, including Saturdays? How often do you find members of the upper echelon at the office on Saturdays?

If it is a Saturday when only your peers will be there, then your clothes can reflect a decidedly casual attitude. After all, you're there to get work done, not to impress anyone (not with your clothes, that is; we will hope that coming in on a Saturday *does* impress someone and works to your advantage). You might wear khaki cotton pants, corduroys, or maybe even well-kept jeans, with a windbreaker or a sweater. A navy blazer is probably dressier than necessary. You could, of course, wear a more brightly colored blazer or a bold tweed jacket. Topsiders, loafers, or maybe even sneakers will do. As for shirts, anything from a brightly colored cotton button-down or tattersall, worn open at the neck, to a knit shirt might be appropriate.

Are you coming in for a meeting, perhaps with an out-of-town customer? If you like to wear suits, and your office frowns on anything more casual than dark, traditional models, the weekend could be your opportunity to wear a tan suit, a seersucker, or a wool tweed. These also could work well if your Saturday involves a lunch date with a customer.

SATURDAY NIGHT:
Cocktail Party with Colleagues

The image you are projecting in this social/business affair is that you are confident and can be social while remaining in control of all elements.

There are distinctly different types of business-related parties. Sometimes the boss is host. Sometimes it is one of your colleagues. Occasionally it is someone who works for you.

If you are concerned with what to wear, *don't* ask the host. You are bound to hear something noncommittal like, "Oh, anything casual." Then you show up in a polo shirt, only to find everyone decked out in posh resort casuals. Avoid that fiasco by asking peers who are also invited what they will be wearing. I know everyone wants to appear cool and not ask. But it is better to sacrifice that one instant of coolness and enjoy the event because you are dressed properly.

Party clothes can be fun and can boost your image in your colleagues' eyes. Your co-workers get to see a whole different you, and you get to show some of the really great clothes you own. You might choose a blazer in camel hair or navy cashmere with a silk handkerchief tucked in the breast pocket, or a subtle silk, linen, and wool tweed sports jacket. An interesting look that is popular today is a boldly patterned sweater. Perhaps your taste runs more to handsome pastel-colored linens or cottons or to the smoother look of colored ultrasuede.

Shirts can run the gamut from a blue dress model with a white contrast collar, collar pin, and French cuffs, to a red- or blue- or yellow-and-white-striped button-down; or from a bright pink shirt to a plaid cotton or even a flannel. I'd recommend a contrast collar only if you know that the others are going to be somewhat dressed up. The flannel shirt can present the opposite problem: You may be far too underdressed unless you know that most of the guests will appear in jeans.

A Safe
Middle Ground

Most of the other combinations just mentioned are safe bets. If you wear any of them with a tie, perhaps a cotton sweater and flannel trousers or cotton khakis, you are on safe middle ground. If the group is more casually dressed than you are, it is the simplest thing to:

- Remove your tie, unbutton the top two buttons of your shirt, and be equally informal.

    If they are even more at ease than that, you can go a step further:

- Take off your jacket and roll up your sleeves one or two turns.

You can't, however, come underdressed and then add these touches. (Slip-on loafers—in good condition—in a versatile shade of medium to dark brown or cordovan will support any of these outfits.)

If you're sure of the tone of the party and the type of guests, you can be a bit more individualistic:

- Wear a bow tie and dress pants with suspenders.
- You might try the patchwork or sailboat motif cotton trousers so popular in Ivy League circles.

Color Rule for Leisure Wear

Pick up—that is, repeat—the least dominant, but still clearly visible, color in a pattern. Use that color for the solid (or plain) color in another piece of your outfit.

An example: a plaid shirt with three colors:
- predominantly blue
- secondarily khaki
- a faint line of yellow

Khaki is the least dominant color in the plaid, but is still clearly visible. Wear khaki pants with the shirt.

Another example: a striped sport shirt that is:
- primarily red
- subordinate stripes of blue
- smaller gray stripes

Wear the shirt with gray pants or shorts. Or choose the exact shade of blue from the shirt as the color of the pants.

Or turn it around and come from the other direction. You have khaki cotton pants. When shopping for a shirt to wear with them, look for a pattern that has two or more colors. One of the colors—but not the dominant one—should be khaki. Notice that the two-color rule of business dress as explained in chapter 9 is relaxed somewhat in leisure wear. Two colors are still smart, but the strong colors of leisure wear can, if unchecked, create too matched-up a look.

The important point to remember when you are deciding which subordinate color to feature is that *it should be the one that can be seen from a distance of six feet or more.* You should not have to hold the garment up close to determine which is the subordinate color. If it can't be seen from a slight distance, the color is too weak. If there are three or more colors in the pattern, your own preference will tell you which of the subordinate colors to work with.

This same color rule works well for layering a shirt and sweater. If the shirt is patterned, choose the least dominant color and select a sweater of that same tone. Or if the sweater is patterned, as an argyle or stripe, find a shirt that is one of the lesser colors in the sweater pattern.

When putting together a two-color combination starting with a pair of white shorts or pants, you can go several routes. You can select a solid color top in:

- red
- bright royal blue
- navy blue
- vivid green

—whatever is your own best color—to contrast sharply with the white. Wearing bold colors is an accepted way for upper-class men to dress when they are not at the office.

However, to put together a combination that really creates a coordinated ensemble based on white shorts or pants, look for a shirt with two or more colors, including white. (Here, we do count white as a color, as in gray and white; yellow and white; or red, white, and blue.)

My strong suggestion is that you avoid what I call the Eastern Seaboard Syndrome: wearing pants too short. All trousers look best with at least a slight break.

Another caution: These clothes work in some circles in some states, but in many parts of the country they are not accepted. Make sure you will not be the odd man out for wearing them.

In addition to pocket squares and brightly colored ties and suspenders, another accessory that adds individuality and works with weekend wear is light-colored and patterned socks. Many pastel argyles and other interesting patterns—herringbones, bird's-eye weaves, cotton or wool socks with "clocks" up the sides, and even plain bright yellow or beige cashmere socks—make for small touches that say "weekend dressing."

SUNDAY:
Golf with the Boss

The image you want to convey here is that you are comfortable—with yourself and with him. Golf clothes are much more flamboyant than those that are accepted elsewhere. Even polyester can creep into the picture. Most golf pants are blends of cotton and polyester; golf sweaters are often blended with acrylic fibers. I'm not suggesting you should shun natural fibers if you prefer them and find them more comfortable. But some synthetics are acceptable. And you can go a little crazy with colors, too. Bright is right here, but keep in mind the principles of good color coordination, even if everyone else on the course tends to look as if he collided with a paint truck.

> If 50 million people say a foolish thing, it is still a foolish thing.
> —BERTRAND RUSSELL

Windbreaker-type light jackets or sweaters are essential on the golf course. They can be made of cotton, wool, alpaca, acrylic, or a blend. Avoid cashmere. It is always soft, luxurious, and beautiful, but generally too warm for the game. Shirts should almost always be made of knitted fabrics, soft and unconfining.

Trousers are best when unadorned, without fancy features. Here is perhaps the one place where beltless trousers are convenient. Or you might wear those that have a soft cotton-webbing belt. Naturally, golf shoes are essential. But just because they are designed to be worn on the fairway does not mean that they have to be white or visible from a thousand yards away. Medium brown or brown and white will do fine.

MONDAY EVENING:
Watching Football on TV at a Local Watering Hole with the Crowd from the Office

You aren't always prepared ahead of time to be dressed perfectly for after-hours lounging. Even if you know ahead of time that you will be going, you don't want to change clothes in a major way to go out drinking; you would look affected if you did: as though you concentrate too intensely on fashion.

If you can plan ahead, and if your day's work schedule permits, dress a little closer to your Friday manner. If you cannot do this, take off your tie and switch your suit jacket to a sweater. It is a good idea to keep a solid basic-color sweater, a burgundy tie (for spot emergencies), and an umbrella at the office.

TUESDAY EVENING:
The Company Softball Game

If the team has a uniform, obviously you'll wear it. If not, shirts can range from a T-shirt with the company logo to a basic workout shirt. As to pants, shorts can lead to scraped knees and shins. You might wear loose jeans, corduroys, sweat pants, or any pants that grass stains won't ruin. A cap and wristbands add to the rakish look, as do sunglasses (especially necessary if you wear contact lenses).

If you are a spectator rather than a player, your appearance on the sidelines could range from the same clothes you wore Monday night (watching football at the local bar) to something far more casual. But remember, you may be sitting on grass.

Your Tuesday night activity might be a workout club, bowling, or another active sport. Obviously, you know the requisite outfit.

Company Box Seats at the Stadium

The image you'd like to project here is that of an interested fan, out for fun and imbued with team spirit. You may have to wear the clothes you wore to work. Perhaps the most important rule governing social and blazer dressing is **never wear a suit jacket as a blazer.**

Try not to wear a pinstripe suit to work that day (unless you are a Yankee fan). A blue suit is okay; a gray suit or a blazer is better. Perhaps a sweater and jacket will be enough to keep you warm.

When you wear a sweater over a shirt, keep the tie on. The look of shirt, tie, and sweater is a good one. But if you decide to wear a sweater with a shirt and no tie, *do not let the collar come outside the sweater.* Shirt collar points should stay inside the sweater, whether it is a V or a crew neck. This is one more advantage of button-down shirts. They make it almost impossible for the collar to misbehave and pop out unattractively.

If you have time to go home and change clothes before the game, you can create a pulled-together, casual look. Cotton khakis or corduroys, cotton shirt, cable-stitched sweater, desert boots, and a lightweight parka might do it.

WEDNESDAY:
Travel to a Conference

Here is where you make it clear that you are sophisticated and worldly. Whether you are traveling first-class, business class, or coach, it is essential to be comfortable, as well as to retain your classic appearance without appearing overdressed.

There are times when your most important contact at the conference begins with a meeting on the plane. Remember what we mentioned in chapter 1 about there being no erase button.

You get only one chance to make a first impression. On the plane, registering at the front desk at the hotel, having a drink in the lobby while your room is made ready—these all are times when you may meet people who are important to you. And they will judge you by your appearance.

The clothes you wear on the plane can be similar to those you might wear on a Friday at the office, but a little more laid back: a navy or tweed blazer, or perhaps a coat over your arm, depending on the weather in both locations, and a dress shirt. A tie is optional. Pleated pants or others that are easy to sit in, or even jeans, are a good look with a tweed sports jacket. Wear comfortable loafers: You may have to do lots of walking through airports.

Always carry a complete outfit on board in case your luggage is lost. One man in my audience told of a time when he was flying to an important job interview. He wore comfortable clothes on the plane: a blazer, gray trousers, a nice blue shirt, and no tie. He arrived on schedule, but his luggage went to another city. He said to me, "Do you know that it is next to impossible to buy a necktie before nine in the morning?" He spent the entire day meeting people who were interviewing him, and he continually began by explaining and apologizing for not having a tie. Predictably, he didn't get the job.

When we start out from a position of disadvantage, we seldom present our best selves. All he really needed was to carry a necktie in his briefcase. Then he would have had one perfect outfit that could have helped him carry the day.

When attending a conference, pack swim wear, golf or tennis clothing, and any other items appropriate for the conference location. Pack for whatever facilities the hotel is said to have. Include your tennis racket or golf clubs, if they are important to you. Take something very casual to wear for breakfast in the hotel: perhaps a warm-up outfit or a rugby shirt and cotton pants. A variety of attractive polo shirts will cover many of these situations, and may even see you through some of the less formal meetings.

Bring along one dressy outfit for dinner at the hotel's rooftop restaurant or one of the area's finer spots. Here you might want to wear a double-breasted medium or light glen plaid suit, with a stylish cotton shirt and tie. Don't forget to pack for the black-tie dinner dance on Thursday evening.

WEDNESDAY EVENING:
Nightclub, Bar, or Dance Club

The pleated pant—the loose look—is a great look for this kind of occasion. You might wear a blazer, an unconstructed jacket, a light-colored sportscoat, maybe even an ultrasuede jacket . . . but not business clothes. Your shirt could range from a fine silk to a linen, from a colorful T-shirt under a jacket (the "Miami Vice" look) to a straightforward oxford button-down. These are best worn without a tie, but you might like the narrow-tie look, the kind you would never wear to the office. Rule of thumb: Choose fewer accessories and jewelry rather than more.

THURSDAY EVENING:
Black-Tie Banquet

Every aspect of black-tie dressing says "elegance." When I speak at conventions and conferences, I am often invited to attend their formal dinner dances. I have never understood what would prompt a man who has arrived at this level of achievement to rent his black-tie outfit for this yearly function. His wife or date is resplendent in her most elegant gown or newest cocktail dress. She wears the finest jewelry she owns (or can borrow), and he comes in a third-rate rental getup.

These cautionary remarks are concerned with renting dinner clothes. Chapter 19 tells you how, when, and why to appear your dashing best in your own dinner jacket.

An excuse that has been offered is that renting a suit when a business function calls for "black tie" is a tax-deductible expense, but buying your own comes out of your own pocket. I am not convinced that such a reason compensates for the position that the wearer puts himself in. Consider that the guests invited to these occasions are the company's best producers. Appearing in someone else's suit makes you look as though you cannot afford your own. It also makes you look like a rookie at formal affairs (they are so rare in your life that you have to rent an outfit). It runs counter to the image that you'd like to project, and makes others wonder if you really do belong there.

If you still need convincing . . .

· Rentals are very expensive. The cost of renting a few times could equal the price of your own well-tailored evening clothes.

· Rentals are almost always made of fabric with a high polyester content; thus, they are warm and uncomfortable. That's especially true when you are dancing.

· A rented outfit never fits correctly. The rental company promises all sorts of individual alterations, many of which they totally ignore. When the clothes are delivered to your hotel on the day of the function, it is too late for you to do anything about the missing alterations. The wearer of an ill-fitting dinner suit spends half the evening tugging and pulling at his jacket and adjusting the collar. Often the shirt doesn't fit well, either. All of this rearranging calls attention to the poor fit and makes it even more obvious that your clothes are rented.

My advice: If formal evenings arise more often than every few years, and you hope or plan to be among those who are invited to attend, it would be a wise investment for you to buy your own set of formal dinner clothes.

If there is one area of men's dress where the rules are conveniently strict and prescribed, it is in black-tie dressing. Whether you call it a dinner suit, evening clothes, formal wear, dinner jacket, black tie, or a tuxedo, it all means the same thing. (The French call this kind of dress *le smoking.*) It all adds up to black and white dressing.

18

Three Walks on
the Casual Side

To avoid the cookie-cutter effect, you can take a current style, base your look on it, and still be very much your own man. If you decide that Armani, Lauren, or Fezza has the look for you, think what touches you might add—or omit—to make it distinctly yours. It needn't be a designer's look at all; it might just be a whole new *approach* to style.

As examples of dressing within a mode, but moving outside a set of rigid rules, let's consider three walks. You are getting ready to spend an afternoon strolling through each of three widely different settings.

First, a crisp fall day in a big city: a visit to a museum, a stop at an espresso bar and then on to a first-run movie. Next, a walk in the country. And third, a stroll from your hotel in Florence, Italy, to the Uffizi Galleries.

In each instance you draw on a core theme. Let's see how you ring variations on those themes, making them distinctly your own.

A Walk in Town

You are on your way to a museum, from there a stop at an espresso bar, and then, if the lines aren't forbidding, to the newest movie.

This is an ideal time to explore the wonderful, if tricky, world of dressing in neutrals. Neutrals are colors that do *not* appear in the rainbow such as white, gray, beige, and khaki.

Only a knowledgeable dresser knows how to work with neutrals. He knows a beige jacket made of camel hair or linen or rough-textured silk is passable and safe when worn with the expected pair of dark brown slacks, but it looks tonier and more sophisticated worn with dark gray trousers. He knows what to do with a tan or khaki suit—how to add a pastel-and-khaki-striped tie—to turn it into a really smashing look.

The World of Neutral Colors

I suggest that you begin with a camel sports jacket and introduce gray slacks for a sophisticated look. They could be almost any shade of gray, but the smartest shade with camel is a dark bankers' gray or even darker charcoal gray. With this, choose a white pinpoint oxford cloth button-down shirt or a very creamy shade of off-white. Either works well.

Black shoes are obviously right with the gray trousers, yet a fine, rich dark brown shoe is more interesting. It emphasizes the brown and gray combination. Add a brown belt to match and the outfit is almost complete.

For the man who knows and loves clothes (and I am hoping that you are fast becoming one of them), let's add the one touch that pulls it all together and turns your outfit into a really terrific look: a sweater. Once again there are simple and obvious choices: a tan or light gray V-neck sleeveless pullover. Either shade would make a good match. A bright

Choosing the **Right** *Sweater*

yellow sweater would work well with the outfit, but that would be an accent color and would move you out of the realm of neutral dressing.

My top choice would be to combine your jacket and trouser colors in an argyle pattern of gray and camel. Argyles do come in those shades, but they are not easy to find. For this look, avoid the usual color choices of blue and green, navy and gray, and burgundy and gray when you are sweater shopping. Look for a sweater with all neutral colors with either a gray background or a camel background. It will be a valuable permanent addition to your wardrobe.

This outfit needs no tie, but you certainly could wear a camel-colored wool or a gray wool tie with it if you like.

A Walk in the Country

What you wear for this walk depends upon the time of year and the weather. In warm weather a pair of shorts, a polo shirt, and sneakers make sense. In early autumn a good combination might start with a navy cotton turtleneck shirt worn under a red plaid cotton flannel shirt. With it you might wear a pair of jeans and a pair of sturdy walking shoes like Bass Weejuns.

As the weather turns colder, you might adopt a black cotton knit shirt under a red brushed cotton or red Viyella (cotton and wool) shirt, all topped with an overscaled red and black lumberjack "buffalo plaid" checked shirt. Wear these with gray cotton corduroy pants, a cap, and a pair of lightweight hiking boots.

For an extra layer of warmth when it is very cold outside, you might wear a super-thin pure silk undershirt. These can be found in ski shops or sporting goods stores. They are not inexpensive, but they are amazingly durable and keep you warm without giving you that bulky feeling that you get when wearing long underwear. They are wonderful for any cold day's activity, even shoveling snow.

A Walk in Italy

From your hotel in Florence, you'll stroll to the incomparable Uffizi Galleries.

Protective Coloration

Europeans look and feel better in clothes that are not overly elaborate. They respect subtlety and classic looks in clothes. They would never wear suit, shirt, tie, shoes, and hat from the same designer. Their interest is in a quiet look that says "elegant."

If you are doing business overseas, it is important to remember that no one is more attuned to dress than a European businessman. (He may not own as many clothes as an American, but each outfit he wears looks terrific.) Never wear brightly colored trousers—the kind that make their way to weekend cocktail parties in Connecticut—and do not wear trousers that are too short.

Your outfit for your walk should be about as sophisticated as you can assemble and still be casually dressed. A perfect casual look might include such elegant sportswear as Roger Baugh's linen and silk cardigan jacket—a softer and less constructed look than a blazer—worn with a linen plaid shirt and linen and wool blend trousers. Or wear a solid-color shirt under a patterned sweater and no jacket. Lately, American boating-type shoes are extremely popular in Europe with casual clothes.

An indisputably classic combination, guaranteed to be accepted, is a navy blazer, powder blue point-collar broadcloth shirt, navy-and-white-striped repp tie, and perfectly tailored gray (or light tan) fine wool gabardine trousers. Wear these with highly polished medium-weight shoes in cordovan or black. If you should be invited to a friend's home for dinner (Europeans are uncommonly gracious to visiting business associates and entertain quite grandly), the same type of outfit is perfect, especially if the shirt has French cuffs.

Some years ago I was in Treviso, a small city north of Venice, on a business trip with my husband. We were taken on a plant visit and out to lunch by the head of the company.

Apparently we impressed Giorgio, our host, because we were then invited to his home for the following evening's dinner. He assured us that it would be quite "simple." I assured my husband, however, that nothing about the dinner would be simple. How did I know? he asked. I said,

"Anyone who shows up in a sporty little Fiat, as Giorgio did, dressed in such a studiedly casual way with smart leather driving gloves and fine shoes to show us around a stone quarry, would not do anything in a simple way. Least of all would he give a 'simple' dinner party."

I also believed I had detected a style peculiar to the region. The style was that of wearing French cuffs open; that is to say, unfastened, without cuff links. My husband, a pretty sharp dresser himself, said that perhaps Giorgio had just forgotten to put them on. I said "*That* man? He would never forget anything in an outfit. No, I'm sure it's the style."

The next evening we arrived at a jewel of an Italian villa. It was decorated entirely with brown velvet furniture. Our host's wife had been a model in Milan; she swept into the room in that distinctive way of walking that models have, looking gorgeous.

Giorgio and two other male guests all wore French-cuffed shirts, devoid of cuff links. My guess was right.

Later I learned the reason for their "lapse." Italian men in that upper social stratum all dressed so absolutely perfectly that, in order not to appear as dandies, they purposely created a mistake in their appearance. In the same way, weavers of the world's finest Oriental silk rugs purposely cast a mistake into the design. Nothing should be too perfect.

Casual Dressing and Its Direct Opposite

I hope you have made a note of the wonderfully varied looks you can achieve through informal dressing: A deliberate emphasis on neutrals, or an outdoorsman's layered look, or a reflection of sophisticated, European styles are three of them.

If you plan carefully the way you will combine elements—there is nothing "casual" about it; no reliance on last-minute tossing together an outfit—you will project an authoritative, "He's right on all occasions" image.

However, certain events require a look that is 180 degrees removed from casual. It is as rigidly predetermined as dressing can be. Black-tie dressing is the mode; and the next chapter answers any hows and whys that might stand between you and the splendor of an exactly right formal appearance.

19

Black-Tie Dressing

Maybe because the jet-set fellers spend so much time in their dinner suits, they treat them as normal gear. . . . The "chic" man wears *very simple* formal wear, while the plumbing salesman at his annual wing-ding pretends he's Errol Flynn.
—From *Man in Charge* by
John Weitz and Everett Mattlin,
copyright © 1974 by John Weitz and Everett Matlin

The Look at a Glance

The suit is always black. The shirt is always white with vertical pleats in front and with French cuffs. (In summer the jacket may be white. All else remains the same.)

Suits are fashioned in one of three different collar and lapel styles: *shawl, peaked,* or *notched*. Lapels are either of *satin*, a silklike, smooth, glossy fabric, or of *grosgrain (pronounced grow'-grain)*, a heavy, ribbed fabric resembling a twill. Grosgrain is also known as *faille* (pronounced *file*).

Along with the three types of lapels, there are two types of closings—*single-breasted* and *double-breasted*. Double-breasted jackets are kept buttoned at all times. A double-

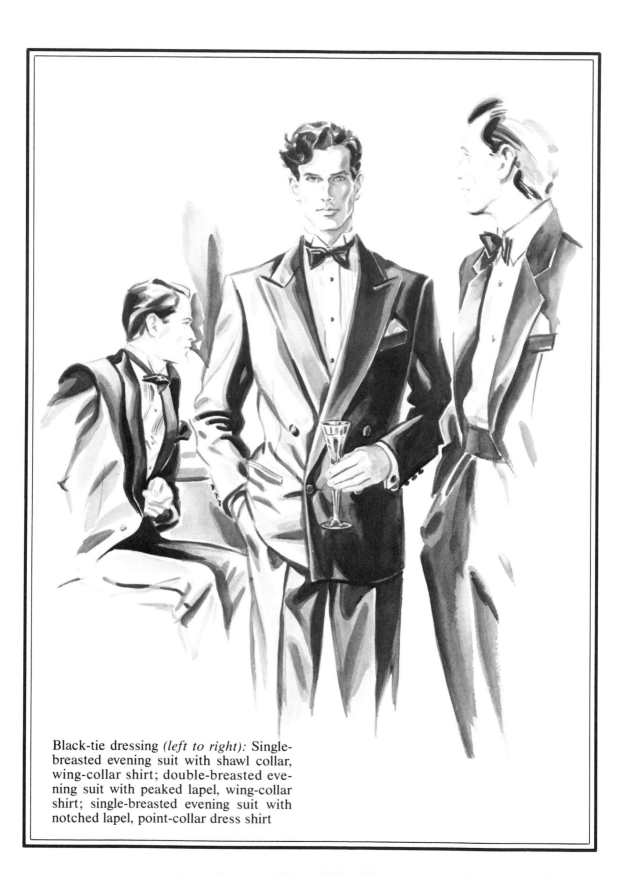

Black-tie dressing *(left to right):* Single-breasted evening suit with shawl collar, wing-collar shirt; double-breasted evening suit with peaked lapel, wing-collar shirt; single-breasted evening suit with notched lapel, point-collar dress shirt breasted model should not be your first and only evening suit, because it will come and go in style. It does, however, have one advantage: It eliminates the necessity to wear a cummerbund. A recent innovation—an all-in-one satin waistband on some formal trousers—is not an ideal substitute for the traditional cummerbund; it looks like what it is, a replacement for the real thing.

Naturally, the trousers of the evening suit match the fabric of the jacket. A ribbon runs down the outside of the trouser leg; it matches the lapel material. Thus, if the suit jacket has a satin lapel, the ribbon down the side of the leg is also satin; or they are both grosgrain.

Another note on the trousers: This is the one time when cuffs are *never* worn. The style of wearing cuffs on trousers originated in England. They were called turn-ups. They resulted from a man's turning up the bottoms of his trousers to protect them from soiling as he walked around his country estate. Accordingly, men wore cuffs on their tweedy suits or country flannels, but not on their formal evening wear.

Penguins, Not Peacocks

In recent years, black-tie dressing has experienced a happy return to its classic style and has moved away from some of the excesses of the recent past: pastel ruffled shirts and a rainbow of colors for the suits.

Only black and white are correct. Only black and white are elegant. Small touches, including colored bow ties, cummerbunds, and pocket squares have become acceptable in limited circumstances; but to be sure, count on black to be right.

Recently I was working with one of the men I counsel on dress, a university president. Since his promotion to president, his need for formal clothes had expanded. We were outfitting him in a second evening suit, one with a notched lapel rather than the shawl collar style he already owned. I told him that his own formal shirt and bow tie were probably fine since these classic items don't change much. But just to be sure, I asked him if perhaps his bow tie was the wider style that had been popular several years earlier but was no longer in style. He said, "No, my bow tie is fine and so is my shirt. It's a nice blue one with ruffles."

"No!" I said. "That's for the bandleader!" We added a new formal shirt to the list of items to buy.

Formal Flair

· **Shirts.** A formal shirt has French cuffs and an unusual button arrangement. Unlike regular shirts, a formal shirt does not come with buttons on one side and corresponding buttonholes on the other. Instead, it is designed with a set of buttonholes on both front edges of the shirt.

When you examine the shirt in the store, it looks as though it buttons normally. In order to package the shirt for retail sales, the manufacturer supplies a ribbon with sewn-on buttons that fit through both sets of buttonholes. When you open the shirt and prepare to wear it, you merely remove the strip of ribbon and the attached buttons, and substitute a set of studs, small pieces of formal jewelry that slip through the buttonholes and act as fasteners.

Formal shirts are *always* worn with cuff links. They should be of simple design, generally matching the studs: gold; platinum; gold plate; opaque stones such as onyx, lapis lazuli, or mother-of-pearl; enamel. Or they might be the newer and inexpensive handsome black silk knots. These latter are available at better stores and sell for about $5 a pair. Many well-dressed Europeans, who often wear evening clothes, favor silk knots over expensive cuff links. It is a crisp, chic look.

A point of current style: The only *totally* correct formal shirt for black-tie dressing is one with a standard type of straight point collar. Wing collars are correctly reserved for "white tie and tails." But the wing collar is so flattering a style that it is currently becoming very popular with black-tie dress—both the conventional black evening suit and the white dinner jacket and black evening trousers worn only in summer months.

· **Suspenders.** Often referred to as "braces" in higher-priced magazines and better stores, suspenders are always worn with formal trousers. Buttons sewn inside the trouser waistband fasten to the suspenders. As with bow ties, avoid the tacky look of clip-on suspenders. (In fact, I cannot think of anything that clips on that is appropriate.) The traditional braces worn with black tie are made of black or white silk. But almost any variation, from bright red cotton to black and white polka dots, is acceptable.

· **Bow Ties** should be made of the same fabric as the lapels of your suit—either satin or grosgrain. They should not be clip-on (too reminis-

SIX EASY STEPS FOR TYING A BOW TIE PROPERLY

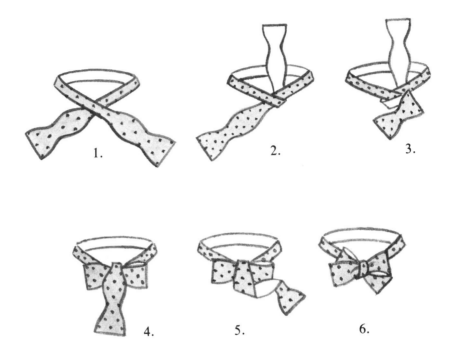

1.   2.   3.

4.   5.   6.

Today more men are choosing the bow tie as a form of personal expression: occasionally for business wear, more often for social situations, and as an essential part of formal dress. Learning how to tie your own bow is only slightly harder than tying your shoe.

1. Begin with one end (whichever one you prefer, but if you are right-handed, it is usually easier to hold the longer end in your right hand) 1½ inches longer than the other. Cross the longer end over the shorter one.
2. Bring the longer end up through from the back. (*This* part is the same as tying your shoe.) Keep long end above the other. Pull tight.
3. Steps 3 and 4 are the crucial ones, *different* from tying your shoe. The original shorter piece is now the one that hangs closest to your body. Form front loop by folding this short end horizontally across (making a sort of S shape exactly as in drawing number 3).
4. While holding front loop, drop long end down in front.
5. Create second loop with it by poking long end through hole behind first loop. This part is once again just like tying your shoe.
6. Pull two parts evenly. Loosen the part around your neck until comfortable. Tighten the bow. This takes some adjusting and practice at first. (It gets easier and is worth the effort to learn.)

Note: When it's finished, a real bow tie (as opposed to the clip-on and some ready-tieds) has a loop in front on one side and an end in front on the other side.

cent of a high school prom) or previously tied (too perfect). By following the diagram and directions on the preceding page, you'll realize that tying your own is easier than you think.

The bow tie is the one item in this classic outfit that seems to vary most with changing times. For a few years the ties are rather narrow; then the style is for them to be wider and a bit floppy. Currently they are narrow once again. It is wise to pay attention to this small point of fashion. Check the men's fashion magazines to see if yours is in style. For an investment of approximately $12, your whole outfit can be brought up to date.

If you are very much on the cutting edge of dressing for excellence and are wearing a wing collar shirt, it is important for you to wear a bow that you tie yourself. It is the only type that has an unbroken band around the neck, all of which is apparent to the viewers.

· **Cummerbunds.** Just as your bow tie matches the fabric of your lapels, so should your cummerbund. The cummerbund is worn with the pleats facing up—originally intended to catch stray crumbs at dinner! Recently a variant of the strict black and white has crept in. Some men are seen wearing colored or patterned matching bow ties and cummerbunds. In the most elegant circles, black and white remains the rule. But if you are in a social set that dresses frequently in formal clothes, then you may be looking for variety. I caution against abandoning the basics, but you might enjoy testing your wings on locally acceptable options.

· **Pocket Squares.** Choose silk in white or in a bright, dashing touch of color, or opt for the always safe and correct white linen handkerchief. Either choice should be placed simply, unobtrusively in your breast pocket.

· **Socks** worn with evening clothes are always black. Ideally, but not necessarily, they are black silk, which are sometimes hard to find. Any black to-the-calf or over-the-calf socks will do. If ever a small flaw could loom large enough to ruin an entire impression, it would be wearing short socks that allow skin to show when you are seated.

· **Shoes.** The correct shoe to wear with formal garb is so far from what most men—particularly young ones—can conceive of wearing that I feel obliged to offer an alternative. The correct formal shoe is a black patent-leather low-cut slip-on with a flat ribbon bow; it is known as a dancing pump. It is lightweight, comfortable, and obviously perfect for dancing.

Evening pumps are special shoes suitable for nothing but formal wear and are thought by the uninitiated to be a bit on the dandy side. Many men whom I have been able to convince to dress in newer, more distinctive ways than they have ever done before still balk at the patent-leather pump. The top-drawer men of the social world, however, who appear superbly and often in formal dress, think of it as perfectly natural.

Nevertheless, some of the executives I dress have chosen to adjust the rule slightly. I tell them that a perfectly plain, black lace-up shoe, patent leather or highly polished, is the nearest acceptable substitute. It is not precisely in the tradition, but no one would be faulted for the change. On the other hand, wearing slip-on loafers of any kind, no matter how highly polished, does not make the grade.

As evening clothes are generally worn at social events with women attending, I'll tell you something you may not know, but should. Like James Bond, every man looks wonderful—debonair, sexy, and in command—when he is in formal attire. Ask any woman.

A Little-Known Bargain

One way around the expense of purchasing a formal evening suit is to visit one of the many "previously owned" shops. Often this is a good place to pick up a wonderful bargain. For any of who-knows-what reasons, dashing dressers bring fine formal clothes to these stores and sell them for a pittance. You can buy them for not too much more.

Occasionally, you may find a 100 percent wool tropical-weight dinner suit for between $50 and $100. Then, after a trip to the best tailor you can find (who may charge you another $50–$70), you have a perfectly fitting, high-quality suit for between $100 and $200. In a department store or speciality shop, such a suit would cost well over $300. Moreover, the older suit may have a variety of small touches—better-grade buttons, a true buttonhole on the lapel, lining in the trousers' knees—that recent cost cutting has prompted manufacturers to eliminate. And you will have had the adventure of discovery. Add your own purchases of a new shirt, tie, and accessories, and you will have a dash of individuality.

20

Questions Most Often Asked of a "Wardrobe Engineer"

I have noticed that certain questions are asked over and over at my Executive Wardrobe Engineering sessions. You may have some of the same concerns, so I will share these frequently asked questions—and the answers—with you. Here is a double handful of them.

Q. You mentioned tipping the tailor. How do I do it? Do I hand him the money or can it be added to my bill?

A. The tip is a personal matter. You cannot have it added to your bill. It is passed in the same way that one normally tips the captain or headwaiter in a fine restaurant—hand to hand. And it should be done discreetly, because officially the tailor in a men's store is not permitted to accept money, although it is done all the time.

Q. How many suits should I have?

A. "How many" is not important. What matters is *how good* each suit looks on you. You may think people remember that you keep wearing the same suits over and over again. That is not true. If you look terrific in the few good suits you own, people will remember that you always look good. If you have five or six mediocre suits, they will remember that you always look ordinary.

Most men have one suit that is the right one for most occasions, the one they can reach into the closet for and count on to be perfect. What you want to do each time you invest in a new suit is to try to find one more that fits into this perfect-suit category. Instead of buying two or three new suits a year, spend a bit more and buy one outstanding one.

Q. What is the least expensive way to give my wardrobe a lift and make two suits look like a whole collection?

A. Buy three or more different shirts for each suit and two ties for each shirt. That gives you at least six different looks for each suit you own. Obviously, this is far less expensive than buying more suits.

Q. How is dressing for an interview different from regular business dress?

A. Interview dressing should be quite conservative. It should send the message that you are not the type to rock the boat, not the type to try to shock anyone or to call unnecessary attention to yourself. Does this sound as though I am suggesting that you dress rather innocuously for an interview? Yes, I am.

After you have passed the first interview and are ready for the second, usually with someone at a higher level, your clothes may express a touch more individuality. But proceed with caution. After you have the job, you may express more of your own personal style. (In interviews careful grooming is crucial. Polished shoes are a must.)

Q. What if everyone else in my office dresses poorly, or at any rate not very well?

A. If that is the case, you're lucky. It won't be hard for you to stand out from the crowd. My advice is: Don't dress for the job you have, but for the job you are aspiring to have. The chief executive does not want to worry whether he'd be embarrassed when dining with you and an important client. Nor does he relish arriving at his club early to tell a third person, "Look, no matter what this fellow looks like, he's really a sharp guy." Don't let others' lack of taste bring you to their level.

Q. Do I have to dress just to impress other people, or can I express myself?

A. Impressing someone is only one reason for selecting certain clothes. There may well be times when you do not want to impress *too* much; not come on too strong in a "powerful pinstripe" suit. On the other hand, when you are out to sell yourself to a potential client or an existing one, you will want to project a professional look. So you will choose a dark, expensive outfit—a power suit. It becomes a powerful form of self-expression conveying nonverbally that you are effective and assertive.

Q. What are the most common mistakes you see in men's appearance?

A. Wearing items of clothing that are too short. The most common mistake is wearing short trousers—ones without a break. This mistake is frequently made by men who are otherwise well dressed. Wearing short-sleeved shirts with business suits is another common error. A short-sleeved dress shirt is a contradiction in terms. Part of what gives a shirt its "finish" is its long sleeves and crisp cuffs. Without those, you have a less polished look.

Wearing socks that are too short and bare part of the leg when a man is seated is a common mistake. Another error is wearing a necktie that is too short. A tie should extend down to the lower edge of the belt buckle.

Did you notice that all of these are "free" improvements? None of them will cost you a cent.

Q. What can I do to make a difference in how I look without going to great expense?

A. 1. Use color well. Color is free. Coordinate your colors skillfully and people will notice.

2. Be well groomed. Polished shoes are free; they just take a bit of time and energy. Get a good haircut, and get it done frequently enough to prevent that newly shorn look. (Haircuts are not free, but not expensive enough to worry about.)

3. You might occasionally wear a collar pin. It is dapper and will instantly "lift" your look, yet the investment is only about $10.

Q. What do I do with some of my older clothes that aren't quite as "with it" as my newer purchases? Is there some way to make them work?

A. Since suit lapels and ties have been changing in width, you probably have an assortment of different sizes in your closet. Combine them carefully. A wide tie will look out of place with a natural-shouldered, medium-lapel suit. Similarly, a wide tie is incompatible with new, fashion-forward designer shirts. And designer shirts certainly don't work with a Brooks Brothers Ivy League suit. It's all a matter of proportion. There is little you can do to fit together dissimilar styles, but as the pendulum of style swings, you may find some of your older purchases returning to favor.

Q. You mentioned "transitional dressing." Could you give a few more examples of how to dress when spanning the seasons?

A. Neckwear is a case in point: It can help you make a smooth transition from one season to the next. If warm, springlike days come along when the calendar says it is winter and you are still wearing winter-weight clothes, you can spring into March with softer, pastel-toned neckties. Moving into fall, on crisp days in September you do the reverse: Wear darker, earth colors, including rusts, maroons, and burgundies, instead of light-colored ties.

Another way is to vary your suiting fabrics. The three weights of suits are lightweight tropicals, ten-month weights, and winter weights. Near the end of the winter season you can hurry spring along by changing to a ten-month weight. The reverse procedure works in early fall or late summer.

Slacks, too, are an agent for transitional dressing. When a warmer season approaches, change from flannels and worsted fabrics to lighter weights and lighter-colored gabardines. As the weather turns cooler, switch from tropicals to lightweight, darker-colored wool gabardines.

Shirts also offer an opportunity to span the seasons. Brooks Brothers has just introduced a new, lighter-weight oxford cloth shirt. It has the traditional appearance, yet the weave of the fabric makes it ideal for summer wear. Similar shirts should be widely available from other manufacturers by the time you read this.

Q. What is a basic business wardrobe?

A. Three to five suits and a navy blue blazer. Add to these a pair of gray slacks and a pair of camel or khaki slacks. This is the core of a man's wardrobe, not necessarily purchased in that order. The navy blazer is the most versatile item in his closet. It is so versatile that it might well be the first item purchased. In a pinch, it will work instead of a suit for job interviews. If I had to choose just one combination with a navy blazer, it would be khaki trousers, a light blue button-down shirt, and a yellow silk foulard tie.

Q. If a blazer is so widely accepted, when can I wear it to work?

A. For every industry and for every company, the rules are different. Many firms, such as those in financial services, require that you wear a suit every day. On the other hand, if you teach or if you work in certain areas of manufacturing, wearing a suit could be overdressing.
Some people in sales must wear suits. Others know that their clients would find a suit too formal. Here is where you must use your own good judgment. And use your eyes. See what others in your industry, in your company, and in your office do.

Q. If I feel I can't buy the best of everything, are there any specific categories where I would do well to concentrate on spending more?

A. A good basic rule is to spend more in three categories: on darker items, on winter items, and on classic items. You can economize—that is, not pay top dollar—on lighter-colored clothes, like a tan poplin suit; on spring or summer clothes, like a lightweight sports jacket; and on an item of clothing you'd like to own just because it is "in" and currently popular, like a straw hat. But a navy pinstripe winter suit, which combines all three "top dollar" categories, should be the best you can buy.

Q. You've convinced me not to wear white shoes. But what shoes should I wear with white slacks?

A. Dark shoes. I know the idea, when you're not used to it, seems strange. But if you wear them and know it's right, you can wear them with confidence. Soon you will notice other well-dressed men doing the same. White bucks are an exception: You can wear them for a casual, Ivy League look.

Q. You have said that medium to dark brown ties are okay, but wearing dark brown suits is not okay. Isn't that a contradiction?

A. Not at all. Dark brown suits are not accepted in fine business circles. The reason is obscure, but accept the fact as a given. Tan suits are a classic. The rule for coordinating suits with shirts and ties tells you to repeat colors, so you would want to wear another shade of brown with your tan suit. Also, as a tie is often darker than a suit, it follows that a medium or dark brown tie works well with a tan suit.

Q. While we are talking about browns and tans, why do you advise that an ivory or cream color is great for a shirt, but that it's best to stay away from beige shirts or tan ones?

A. An ivory or cream-colored shirt is one of the most difficult to find, but it is worth looking for. It should be the color of French-vanilla ice cream, a color that is both elegant and gives rich tone to your skin.

Some people look pale in pure white shirts and are not at their best in them except in the summer, when they are tanned. But a fine cream-colored shirt is always flattering and highly versatile as well.

Tan, ecru, or beige shirts—which are several shades darker brown than cream or ivory—look muddy and unclean. Although the actual difference in hue is slight, the *perceived* difference, when the shirt is against your skin, is tremendous.

Q. What about gray or brown-and-white-striped shirts?

A. All of the problems inherent in beige or tan shirts are also true of medium and dark gray shirts. Extremely light, pearl gray shirts, though, are almost as desirable as ivory or cream ones.

An exception to darker brown or gray shirts' undesirability is the striped shirt. A narrow brown line on a white shirt makes a handsome adjunct to tan suits and brown tweed sports jackets. The same is true for gray stripes on a white ground. This type of shirt is perfect for all of your gray suits and works well with gray tweed jackets. It is the perfect foil for a red or burgundy tie.

Q. When is a jacket worn buttoned, when is it left open, and how does this apply to double-breasted jackets?

A. A single-breasted jacket is worn buttoned when you are standing and open when you are seated. Watch the "Tonight Show" and you will see that when a male guest walks out onto the set, his jacket is buttoned. Just as he sits down, he reaches to unbutton it. One of the advantages of a single-breasted jacket is that it *can* be worn open, too, for a more casual look.

A double-breasted jacket is always worn buttoned. That can be one of its disadvantages—it doesn't look right when it is open. That also is part of its more formal appearance.

Q. Let's say a man wears fine clothes, well tailored and of high quality. He is well groomed. Are there any small points that still can ruin the whole effect?

A. Yes. One that I notice in particular is wearing sideburns that are too long. I know a man who wears $900 Oxxford suits, beautifully made shirts, and expensive shoes. But his sideburns come down to his ear-lobes. It gives him a dated, 1960s look. And that one little point is incongruous with his look of excellence. Sideburns should not be lower than the middle of a man's ear.

Another effect that damages an image of excellence is wearing tinted glasses. I don't, of course, mean sunglasses. I mean tinted prescription glasses. Unless your eyes require them, I would advise against them. Anything that keeps colleagues and clients from being able to establish strong eye contact with you is not a plus.

Q. I have seen many men wearing shirts with rounded collars. What do you think of them?

A. I don't like them, because they resemble the round collars on school uniforms. It is not a masculine look, except when worn with a collar pin. If you like the small-collar effect, try wearing a shirt with a tab collar. It is elegant, has the precision of a pin collar, but, as no hardware shows, it has the advantage of simplicity.

Q. What is your opinion of dress shirts and ties with designers' initials or logos?

A. I think discerning men who dress in good taste avoid logo over-kill. They do not wear shirts or ties bearing another person's initials. Bottega Veneta, a manufacturer of some of the world's finest leather goods, has no visible identification on its products aside from their intrinsic good design. Their slogan is: "When your own initials are enough."

I don't feel nearly as strongly about logos on sports clothes. Sometimes they are hard to avoid. So many really fine casual clothes bear that little polo player or the well-known alligator. They have become an accepted part of our society. If you feel strongly enough against them, you can eliminate them from your wardrobe. But their colors are so wonderful that they are hard to resist.

Q. On some shirts' button-down collars, the collar is pulled taut to the buttons. I have seen others on which the collar has a slightly puffy roll. Which style is right?

A. A button-down collar is by definition a soft, somewhat relaxed collar. It was originally designed as a sport shirt with the points buttoned down to prevent flapping in the player's face. The soft "roll" is an essential part of the look.

Q. How often should I have my suits cleaned?

A. Many American men have their clothes dry-cleaned too often. Certainly I'm not suggesting that you should be anything less than meticulous. But it is important to remember that clothes made of natural fibers do not thrive on an excess of dry-cleaning fluids. When you dress for business each day, you shower, use deodorant, put clean underwear on your clean body and then a clean shirt on top of that. Over all these clean clothes, you wear a suit. Under normal circumstances, barring spots, your suit will remain clean and fresh. If you air out the suit after each wearing, occasionally give it a good brushing, and don't wear it for two days consecutively, there is no need for frequent dry cleaning.

If you own several suits, you will be able to let them "rest" a few days between wearings. Natural fibers are resilient. A good suit will "hang out" and come back to shape. It probably won't need pressing between wearings. If you follow these suggestions, a couple of cleanings during a season should be enough.

Q. How can I take care of my shirts and make them last longer?

A. Shirts should not be heavily starched. The more starch, the more fibers break down, causing the collar and cuffs to fray. Light starch, if you like starch at all, is better for your shirts. If your shirts are hand laundered, the best technique is to use no starch on the body of the shirt and apply spray starch lightly on the collar and cuffs during ironing.

Q. What about ties, shoes, and socks?

A. About *ties,* there isn't much I can tell you except to eat carefully and use Goddard spray on oil-based or grease spots. Other spots are harder to work with. Of course, if you should become a bow tie wearer, you will have an advantage: Your tie will rarely get splashed.

Shoes, like suits, should not be worn two days consecutively. They need time to air out. Cedar shoe trees, when placed in shoes, will absorb moisture from within; keeping them polished will help protect your shoes from rain and rough treatment.

Socks—wool, cashmere, or cotton lisle—ideally should not be machine-washed or -dried. Hand washing and flat drying are best. If this is impossible or impractical, then machine-wash them, but allow them to dry lying flat or hung over a rod. The dryer destroys elastic tops and shortens the life of socks. It may shrink them as well.

One basic rule for longer life in your clothes is to separate laundry into three piles: *Wash all whites together, wash all reds together, wash all other colors together.* Perhaps you will do a load of reds only once a month, but don't make the mistake of sneaking one red item in with your whites. Your favorite shirt could emerge as a pale shade of pink; it is more likely to come out a splotchy rose color.

21

A Final Word

In the first few pages of this book, I made several promises to you. Some were about specific aspects of dressing for excellence; others expressed in general terms the heightened confidence and sense of accomplishment you would experience as you joined the circle of executive whose appearance says "Power." All the facts, as well as the reasoning that underlies them, are in the chapters you have read.

The focus now is on you. Have you begun to notice things that you had overlooked before you became involved with improving your appearance? For instance, have you found yourself evaluating the pattern match at the seams of a colleague's glen plaid suit?

Or how your co-workers dress for an evening or weekend social gathering? Do you notice and appreciate skillfully chosen combinations of suit, shirt, and tie?

You are very much aware of these things not simply because you now know their importance, but because you are skilled at dressing well, and it gives you a new-found source of pleasure.

I have seen this happen over and over again with my clients. After a period of following my lead, a client will soon begin to put together his own combinations—built around, say, a splendid new Bengal striped shirt. I can see him visibly react positively to the harmony—and fun—of it. Dressing for excellence becomes an art form, and you become the artist.

There is another benefit to mastering this art form. If you know you look good, you can get on with other things in life. You can focus attention and energy on what you are doing with the people around you; there's no doubt that you have their confidence and that your suggestions will be taken seriously.

In short, you have an edge of influence when you dress well. At times, it is almost imperceptible, operating beneath observers' level of awareness. *But they feel it,* and they act accordingly. At other times, it is a definite, recognizable aura, and the vote of confidence you win is equally strong.

You have invested dollars and hours to read this book. Why, instead of using your time and money in any of a dozen other ways, have you chosen to learn how to *Dress for Excellence*? Boil it all down, and it's because you want to look like a CEO. My last word to you addresses that point directly: Of course you cannot make it into the inner circle of leaders solely because of your new, authoritative image, but having it is one more way to demonstrate that you are fully at ease in that role. I am delighted if I have been able to help you in this regard. I wish I could share the pleasure and some of the excitement you are going to experience as you move into the company of those who *Dress for Excellence*.

Appendix
Useful Information

SIZE EQUIVALENTS

	SMALL	MEDIUM	LARGE	XL
Sweaters & Sports Clothes				
Shirt Sizes	14½	15, 15½	15½/34, 35 16, 16½	16½/34, 35, 36 17+
Jacket & Suit Sizes	36, 37	38, 39, 40	41, 42	43, 44+
Trouser Sizes	28, 29, 30	31, 32, 33, 34	35, 36, 37	38+

Note: You might want to make a copy of this page and give it to the person (or, if you're lucky, persons) who buys you gifts.

A Comparison of British, American, and Continental Clothing Sizes

SUITS AND OVERCOATS	American	36	38	40	42	44	46	48
	British	36	38	40	42	44	46	48
	Continental	46	48	50	52	54	56	58
SHIRTS	American	14	14½	15	15½	16	16½	17
	British	14	14½	15	15½	16	16½	17
	Continental	36	37	38	39	41	42	43
SHOES	American	7½	8½	9½	10½	11½	12½	13½
	British	7	8	9	10	11	12	13
	Continental	41	42	43	44	45½	47	48
SOCKS	American	—	10	10½	11	11½	12	13
	British	9½	10	10½	11	11½	12	12½
	Continental	39	40	41	42	43	44	45
GLOVES	Sizes are the same							

Foreign Language Translations on Labels

English	COTTON	WOOL	LINEN	SILK
Italian	COTONE	LANA	LINO	SETA
French	COTON	LAINE	LIN	SOIE
German	BAUMWOLLE	WOLLE	LEINEN	SEIDE

Index

*Page numbers in italics denote illustrations. Page numbers in bold face denote charts.